Independent Advocacy and Spiritual Care

Geoff Morgan

Independent Advocacy and Spiritual Care

Insights from Service Users, Advocates, Health Care Professionals and Chaplains

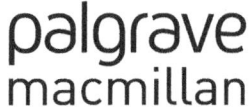

Geoff Morgan
North Middlesex University Hospital NHS Trust
London, United Kingdom
Oxford University Hospitals NHS Foundation Trust
Oxford, United Kingdom

ISBN 978-1-137-53124-7   ISBN 978-1-137-53125-4   (eBook)
DOI 10.1057/978-1-137-53125-4

Library of Congress Control Number: 2016957533

Cover image © Brian Jackson / Alamy Stock Photo
Cover design by Henry Petrides

Printed on acid-free paper

This Palgrave Macmillan imprint is published by Springer Nature
The registered company is Macmillan Publishers Ltd.
The registered company address is: The Campus, 4 Crinan Street, London, N1 9XW, United Kingdom

Foreword

When, as a Justice Minister, I was taking the Mental Capacity Act (MCA) through Parliament, it was met with a wall of opposition—from churches of all denominations, much of the right-wing media and an angry alliance of other groups. I can remember the *Daily Mail* publishing a scaremongering article about the bill under the headline 'Killing the vulnerable.'

Ten years on, the value of the MCA is now widely recognised. I still receive letters from people around the country grateful for how easy the provisions of the Act made it for them to take care of an elderly or highly vulnerable relative.

This is exactly what the Act was designed to do. It was a forward-looking piece of legislation that took into account Britain's ageing population and the fact that one in three people born in this generation will develop dementia later in life. It recognised the difficulties at the time in ensuring that those who lacked mental capacity were properly and fairly represented.

By nature, many of those who do not have full mental capacity are unable to campaign on their own behalf, and so it can be easy for lawmakers to overlook their specific concerns and needs. That is why I believe it is so important that our leaders make a concerted effort to understand the needs of those who are particularly vulnerable, especially those who may be unable to speak for themselves, and take action accordingly. We must ensure that those unable to represent themselves are not denied a voice.

Representation, of course, is something that many of us take for granted. Most people have someone looking out for them who is in a position to stand up for them when needed, whether that is a relative, a teacher, a social worker, a carer or a politician. But life has a way of being unpredictable, and sometimes factors out of our control take away our ability to make our own decisions. There are many—too many—in our society who live with dementia, who struggle with severe learning disabilities, or who have suffered a brain injury, severe mental health condition, stroke or sudden accident and who, through no fault of their own, have become incapable of making their own decisions.

It had previously been unclear who was responsible for the welfare of these individuals, but the MCA changed this. It helped ensure that those with reduced mental capacity were properly taken care of. Usually this meant help from an appropriate relative or friend, who was given legal power over their affairs, but there was also provision in the Act for the appointment of independent advocates who would represent someone lacking mental capacity. It ensured that those who are unable to represent themselves always have someone on their side, fighting for them and ensuring they receive the same level of representation as the rest of us.

The MCA also empowers individuals when it comes to their future care, through the establishment of a system of advance statements and decisions. Commonly referred to as living wills, individuals were given the power to write down their preferences, beliefs, and values when it comes to their future care, creating documents that provide personalised guidance and insurance to carers should the individual lose capacity at some point later in life.

The Act enshrined a set of principles and safeguards to ensure that carers and health professionals are following a proper procedure when making decisions on behalf of another person. It clarified what was meant by mental capacity, and how to assess whether or not someone had it. Prior to this Act, health professionals were given the difficult task of determining who lacked mental capacity, without the adequate tools necessary to make these judgements. The central tenet of this legislation is to provide health professionals and carers with a streamlined two-stage test to determine an individual's capacity.

Together, these measures transformed the lives of many vulnerable people in Britain and made it easier for those looking after them. This Act had a very real impact on some of the most vulnerable people in our country, protecting them from abuse and ensuring the fundamental right of every person to make his or her own decisions.

Of course, that is not to say things cannot improve further. While the MCA has provided a solid foundation for treatment of those who lack mental capacity, there have been obstacles when it comes to its implementation. There remain concerns that care workers and vulnerable people lack a fundamental understanding of the tenets of the Act and the protections it offers them. We must do more to ensure that the strong principles outlined in the Act are understood by professionals and patients alike and that these principles are continually put into practice.

This book is an important work on a significant piece of legislation. The more this kind of legislation is understood, the more the rights and needs of those whom it concerns will be featured in our national debate, and the harder it will be for these hard-fought rights to ever be withdrawn. I congratulate Geoff on this book.

David Lammy
London, UK
December 2015

Preface

This book explores the profession of independent advocacy by considering its history, and commenting on live examples from practice in London, UK, during the period 2007–2012. Recent relevant changes included the Health and Social Care Act 2012 (especially Sections 67 and 68), the House of Lords Select Committee on Deprivation of Liberty Safeguards (DoLS), the Cheshire West judgement, post-legislative scrutiny of the Mental Health Act (MCA) 2007, and amendments under the Care Act 2014. These pinpointed the roles of independent advocates as they widened in importance. This chronology will be covered briefly, but the primary focus of the book is on the *advocate as practitioner* in relation to the service-user, and in offering reflection upon that. The exploration will give the reader an insight into what independent advocates actually do, whether Independent Mental Capacity Advocates (IMCAs), Independent Mental Health Advocates (IMHAs), or professional or generic advocates, figures who now cast increasing light on the British health and social care scene. The book is aimed at advocates and health and social care professionals, lawyers, psychologists, chaplains or spiritual care practitioners, and to ministers of religion, whether from synagogue, church or mosque, on account of its philosophical and theological approach.

Independent advocates are not lawyers. With deference to the latter profession, they are ordinary people trained to support individuals to make choices, take decisions and secure rights in health, social care and housing. However, I found that some very good advocates also have law degrees. Independent advocating activities, which occur both statutorily and non-statutorily in England, may take place on an instructed or non-instructed basis, depending on whether individuals have, or lack, capacity (intellectual ability) to make certain practical decisions, such as a move into residential care, or about serious medical treatment such as having a feeding tube inserted, or treatment for cancer.

The emergence of statutory independent advocacy from occupation to profession is one which I have found fascinating to be in the middle of as a practitioner. Measures have been applied and debates have taken place in relation to the training needs of advocates. In order to establish its distinctiveness, advocacy has sometimes been associated with more developed professions, such as social work and mental health nursing, but here I innovatively connect it with that of the spiritual care giver, in this case the healthcare chaplain. I purposefully use the established disciplines of Practical Theology and Professional Studies to achieve this.

In so doing, I also want to make up what I perceive to be a deficit in the spiritual discourse around health and social care. I argue for its prima facie existence (that spirituality be recognised as a given) in discerning links between theology, spirituality and advocacy practice. This can add qualitatively to the debate about the professionalisation of advocacy because it views advocacy practice alongside Practical Theology in order to see advocacy through the lenses of faith or spirituality. I recognise that there are assumptions here which some readers will reject outright but I also suggest that the view I take of history and practice is sociologically revealing as a slice of life, whether a spiritual angle is accepted or not.

The book signposts and seeks connections, as advocacy itself often does, within independent voluntary organisations and the public sector, between advocacy and patient and public involvement, aspects of philosophy and personal, spiritual and theological development. In case studies and examples, the voices of the 'actors,' from participants I both interviewed (*indicated by italics*) and constructed from literature, are heard. Creative, critical conversations with advocates, their stories and their views on policies are staged, including observations from my professional experience in the advocacy sector. What results yields proposals for enhanced theory, training and practice in independent advocacy and has additional theoretical and practical benefits for those engaged in spiritual care. I invite the reader to use Appendix 2, a list of key questions I used in fieldwork, as a compass on their way through, since I will also refer to these in structuring the guide.

Permissions

I am grateful to the Bethlem Museum of the Mind, Bethlem Royal Hospital, Monks Orchard Road, Beckenham, Kent BR3 3BX, for permission to reproduce 'Melancholia and Raving Madness.'
©BethlemGallery and Museum.

Acknowledgements

Firstly, and most importantly, my gratitude goes out to the 'cast of characters,' the participants without whom this book would have been impossible. Self-advocates and service-users, chaplains and/or spiritual care coordinators, thank you for agreeing to be interviewed. I pay tribute to you and want to celebrate the difference you choose to make in health and social care.

Secondly, I want to say thank you for other support, including some funding, which helped with the project. Specifically, to the (former) Commission for Patient and Public Involvement in Health and the Patient and Public Involvement Forum support organisations, the advocacy schemes, and the NHS where I am currently employed as a chaplain and service manager. In addition, I was grateful for funding from the Continuing Ministerial Education budget of the Anglican Diocese of London.

I am most grateful to the Rt. Hon. David Lammy, MP, for agreeing to pen the Foreword, and for highlighting the enduring value of UK Mental Capacity Act legislation. Dr. Peter Duncan and Prof. Pete Ward, erstwhile Department of Education and Professional Studies of King's College London, were supportive and rigorous in their constructive criticism earlier and ensured, by their encouragement and good humour, that the story was told as cogently as possible.

To my family, friends and colleagues, you have been subjected for a longer time than I had wished to the fall-out from the bouts of writing. I thank you for your kindness, forbearance, accompaniment and love over the time it has taken.

As the Canadian singer/activist, Bruce Cockburn, furiously sang,

> 'I want to raise every voice, at least I've got to try.
> Situation desperate, echoes of the victims cry.
> If I had a rocket launcher... (*Stealing Fire*, 1984),

my hope is that the outcome of this attempt to set out a theological account of independent advocacy will be to 'Raise every voice!' May it result in the greater public good through the mutual enrichment of the practices, on the one hand, of advocacy itself and, on the other, of spiritual and pastoral care!
November 2016

Geoff Morgan
North Middlesex University Hospital NHS Trust
London UK
Oxford University Hospitals NHS Foundation Trust
Oxford UK

Contents

List of Figures

List of Tables

1

Setting the Scene: Who Cares? Why Independent Advocacy Matters

Having been knocked unconscious when his flat is robbed, Liam Pennywell revisits the neurologist who treated him. In her novel, *Noah's Compass*, Anne Tyler recounts how the retired teacher wants to know why his only memory of the attack is waking up in hospital. Supposing the possible perpetrator may be a family member, Liam needs to know from the doctor if he will *ever* recall what happened. While awaiting his appointment, he sees an apparently confused man, supported by a woman. She intrigues Liam. He tells Dr. Morrow that he wishes he had 'someone like the rememberer' out in the waiting room. Realising what Liam means, Dr. Morrow concedes that we could all use a rememberer 'after a certain age' (Tyler 2010, pp. 62–63).

Turning to another kind of story, this time tragically true, David Askew, a 64-year-old man with learning disabilities lived in Greater Manchester, UK. At the beginning of March 2010, he had a heart attack and died when tackling marauding youths, after years of being 'tormented' by them.[1] In

---

[1] David's name joined a tragic litany of names including Steven Hoskin, who was a victim of 'mate-crime,' and those of Francecca Hardwick and Fiona Pilkington, a case which made headlines when a disabled woman died with her mother, who had both been victimised, after which the mother set

© The Author(s) 2017
G. Morgan, *Independent Advocacy and Spiritual Care*,
DOI 10.1057/978-1-137-53125-4_1

the words of David's neighbours, it was like 'bear-baiting.' Events such as these have routinely troubled the UK social conscience. From a human and moral point of view, one felt incensed, impotent, sickened, betrayed. Questions were asked whether police or neighbours could be complicit in these disability hate crimes (BBC-News 2011; Riches 2010, March 12; R. Williams 2010). One issue arising may be what an independent advocacy service could have done to prevent this, and other public outrages, not to mention any kind of approach from the angle of pastoral care.[2]

The above accounts profoundly suggest the need for greater social cohesion, and a stronger safety net, and, I suggest, one means to that end is to draw down the spiritual and theological resources of advocacy. This net is furthermore something that each of us requires. If you haven't personally arrived there yet, at a certain point in life's journey, I have a feeling that, as Dr. Morrow's patient does, you may require another human being in order simply to survive. This support would hopefully come from family or friends. But what if it happens that you don't, or no longer, have family or friends to speak of? Whether it is down to dementia, a physical or learning disability, poor mental health, a history of substance misuse, an acquired brain injury or a safeguarding situation, whatever it may be, don't you have a right to expect the health and social care system to swing in to help you out? How this happens will usually be through informal channels, or by means of friends.

But shouldn't a caring and civilised society consistently ensure that those who are vulnerable and without any other means of support are able to live safely and are not harmed on account of their vulnerability? Shouldn't we guarantee that they benefit from a comforting and practical presence, from someone who can advocate effectively on their behalf? Independent advocacy has an increasingly dynamic part to play (especially after the Care Act 2014 in the UK) in this social safeguard, and I am honoured and privileged to have experienced by what means this has worked out for a few people who could not have survived without it.

---

the car on fire. Failure to defend David from persecution was later classified as 'police misconduct.'

[2] From a different national setting, a front page story in February 2010 noted that Google bosses were convicted in Italy for permitting a mobile phone video, showing the abuse of a boy with Down syndrome, to be posted on the internet in 2006. It was partly through an advocacy group, *Vivi Down*, that the complaint was brought to the Italian court (Prigg 2010).

1   Definition of Advocacy

So what exactly is advocacy, and why does, and should, it matter? This book explores the emerging profession of independent advocacy with regard broadly to spiritual insights from often, but not solely, Christian theology, and by drawing in additional philosophical strands. As a working definition, 'independent advocacy' consists of services staffed by volunteers, or professionals from voluntary or non-profit organisations, commissioned in England or Wales, by local authorities and in relation to Clinical Commissioning Groups (CCGs), formerly known as primary care (or health) trusts. The roles of these advocacy practitioners are then variously to support some individuals to make choices, take decisions and secure rights in relation to health, social care and housing. This activity, which occurs both statutorily and non-statutorily, may take place on an 'instructed' or 'non-instructed basis,' depending on whether individuals, who exclusively have no other means of support, lack capacity to make certain of these above-referenced decisions.

The book carries a number of themes which I shall develop, all of which have a number of dimensions which will appeal to different readers. Firstly, independent advocacy, a newly arrived adjunct occupation in health and social care, has advanced in importance without a thoroughgoing view being taken both of its nature, namely, its changing status into a profession, as well as of the related pressures inherent in such a project. Secondly, this story should be told with reference to a discipline related to the area of pastoral studies, based on the training religious ministers receive, namely—and for those who may be surprised, this is not a contradiction in terms—'Practical Theology'! Thirdly, not much analysis of the role of the independent advocate has been carried out, and even less so by a trained advocate. This is changing of late but there has been little reflection from a spiritual and cultural perspective, even in recent helpful guides. I think here of the contemplative space Independent Mental Capacity Advocate (IMCA) colleagues occupied (without largely religious perspective) as they would take time out to light a candle for a client with whom they alone had spent the last moments of life (M. Graham 2015; K. Newbigging et al. 2015). The picture taken here will draw on questions and, to a lesser extent, on the identification of emergent themes from conversations which I had with various practitioners and service-users.

The book is unique in triangulating voices of advocates, their clients and spiritual care coordinators or chaplains as they speak on the subject of advocacy practice and comment on each other's views. The inherent assumptions of advocacy, as explained briefly above, that this is simply what one human being does for another, may not adequately account for the relationship between the 'tradition' of advocacy and what may be described as the philosophical and theological foundations of what is held out by many as the 'advocacy movement.'

Indeed, in the Western European cultural context, independent advocacy practice can usefully be seen to derive from spirituality, and from Christian faith-based models in particular. This should not undermine the influence of other major religious or philosophical traditions in the broader field—for example, how versions of Buddhism have related well with psychology through the uptake of mindfulness-based therapies by service-users or professionals. Nor does it deny the desire to distinguish the human rights basis of progressive advocacy from some of the perceived negatives of institutional religion—for example, paternalism and social conservatism. I found it useful therefore to draw on Practical Theology, as well as on chaplaincy, which occupies a multi-faith domain, in order to understand the complexity of advocacy practice. The discipline of Practical Theology, in which this book sits, connects appropriately, due to some similarities between the occupations, that of the advocate with that of the chaplain, or 'spiritual care coordinator.' This theoretical foundation will be gently explored historically in the third and fourth chapters. I suspect that there is evidence that independent advocacy, along with some forms of social and pastoral work, is a deeply practical and intensely spiritual or moral, if not religious, function—namely, that it is 'religious' in the broadest Durkheimian definition of the term. For the social scientist Durkheim, religion was a phenomenon which 'bound' an individual or a society to the *sacred* in some way (from Latin *religare*—to bind), and this led me to pursue such an analysis, drawing on certain selected philosophical and theological traditions (B. Turner 2010, pp. 76–7).

2 Approaches Including Practical Theology

One of the chosen methods behind this book is 'explanation-building.' This is a 'strategy of inquiry' in which cases are considered—for example, a programme, event, activity, process, or, as in this particular story, where one or more individuals are covered in depth. 'Bound by time and activity… detailed information (is gathered) using a variety of data collection procedures over a sustained period of time' (Stake cited in Creswell 2009, p. 13; Yin 2006). I had mutual (or creative) critical conversations[3] with my participants, an approach drawn from the discipline of Practical Theology. I also drew on the Critical Realism school and virtue ethics, filters supported by neo-Aristotelian thinkers such as MacIntyre (1985, 1999). These provided access both to one type of 'independent advocacy' tradition and to a means to expand and then develop a more functional synthesis of the model. This development is based on themes from the engagement with participants, service-users, advocates and others who agreed to be interviewed.

This book is original for three reasons: in the fact that independent advocacy is significantly under-researched, in the examination and explanation of the topic using a theological and philosophical lens, and in drawing the 'professionalisation of advocacy' into the realm of theology.

The brief definition of advocacy given above will be expanded further in Chap. 3 and cumulatively as part of the rolling review of sources for this book. My experience of this occupation was gained while I was both employed full-time by advocacy organisations in the years 2005–2011 and active as a part-time student. The questions, which I have placed, for those more interested in method, in Appendix 1, provide bases for further professional and thoughtful exploration by readers. For me, they

---

[3] Tracy's (1996) mutual critical correlation model, in which he encouraged interaction between what he called 'Christian facts,' such as 'symbols, texts, images and events,' and human scientific disciplines (Tracy 1996, pp. 22ff., 64) was re-described by Pattison (2000) as a 'creative critical *conversation*' between:

(a) one's own ideas, beliefs, feelings, perceptions and assumptions;

(b) beliefs, perceptions and assumptions arising from the Christian community and tradition;

and (c) the contemporary situation, practice or event which is under scrutiny (Pattison 2000, p. 230).

grew out of the quest to generate new knowledge in relation to advocacy. I wished to deploy philosophical and theological resources in order to set the premises of these disciplines alongside a range of assumptions. Connections with advocacy were founded on its generally perceived humanitarian and human rights-based function and purpose. A Critical Realist approach, deriving from Roy Bhaskar's quest for epistemological space for the transcendent, does not disparage but encourages spiritual perspectives within philosophy and is a useful container both for advocacy studies and Spirituality Studies (Archer et al. 1998; Bhaskar 2002a; A. Wright 2012). Wolfteich viewed the latter as a 'partner' of Practical Theology, and it is one which I will take account of in the story.[4]

It is also necessary to define what I mean by Practical Theology. Primarily I would like it to be the setting for the advocacy story and a *conduit* through which the story can flow into other disciplines. In training programmes for Christian ministers of religion, what is generally called 'pastoral theology' traditionally represents the taught module for initiation (or baptism), marriage and funeral rites for parishioners ('hatch, match and dispatch'). In the last 20 years, Practical Theology became the preferred term for this—and for priestly in-service training—since, firstly, it implied that theology was not only to do with the pastoral 'flock' (eds. Pattison and Woodward 2000, p. 2) but also included wider secular concerns. Secondly, Practical Theology was connected with the 'practice' of the priest/pastor, who was also typically influenced in her or his overall training by modules on psychology and sociology as part of that 'practical' theology. Indeed, the term Practical Theology (in the sense that 'all theology should be practical') has a much richer pre-history in philosophical and classical theology. This has been resurrected for pastoral benefit by Oden (1994), but space precludes coverage of the detail here (Oden 1994; Maddox 1991).

---

[4] 'Spirituality' is defined inclusively, Wolfteich maintained, citing an encyclopedia which included 'Christian, Jewish… Confucian, African… and secular spiritualities' in its volumes ("Preface to volumes: World spirituality: an encyclopedic history of the religious quest" 1986). In the general description in the preface to the series, the 'spiritual core' is described as 'the deepest center of the person… open to the transcendent dimension' (Wolfteich 2012, p. 333). Having become familiar with and used vocabulary typical in this domain, e.g. the Spiritual Dimension of Advocacy, in this full study I am being more particular in terms of disciplinarity and remain within the parameters of Practical Theology (Morgan 2010).

Ballard and Pritchard (1996) and Whyte (1987) described the 'Church's life' as not only related to its self-understanding and grasp of faith, but to changes in society. Thus Practical Theology is also 'triadic, concerned with the inter-relationship of faith, practice and social reality and is aware that the lines of force flow in both directions' (Ballard and Pritchard 1996, p. 18). The practicality of this dual carriage-way, whereby faith-based overtake secular concerns, or vice versa, is emblematic of the way that theology belongs (or arguably should belong) to the traffic of the public sphere. Practical Theology can therefore have normative force in relation to this new consideration of independent advocacy, as I show in the links which I make between advocacy and spirituality. To change the metaphor from traffic to conversation or a concert, I will characterise 'voices' for the interaction with participants, whether clients, advocates or chaplains. The dynamism of these exchanges is actually increased against this sounding board or within the 'auditorium' of the literature of health and public policy, advocacy, personal communications and theology.

To develop this interface between the human sciences and theology further, Browning (1991) had redefined the nature of Practical Theology, following Farley's (1983) impact in locating its trajectory outside the 'clerical paradigm,' in order to provide 'critical reflection on the church's ministry to the world' (Browning 1991, p. 35). This took the focus off the priest, or the chaplain, as sole agents of practical care and spiritual change (Farley 1983). Non-clerical narratives or experiences from youth work, spiritual accompaniment, mental health practitioners or volunteers testified to the expansion of the reach of Practical Theology (Gilbert 2008; Green and Christian 1998; Shepherd 2009; P. Ward 1995).

Alongside this, in a separate historical dimension which affirmed theology cross-cutting into psychology, the influence of psychological and psychotherapeutic models on theology in developments in pastoral care and counselling made itself felt. The overlap between psychology and theology, which the psychiatrist and lay medical missionary Frank Lake brought to the UK in the 1960s and 1970s, was evidence of this. Lake achieved this by means of seminar-based courses on psychiatry for clergy—and what became known as 'Clinical Theology.' In many ways Clinical Theology was an early 'Practical Theology' for the health sector, a dynamic way of understanding and contextualising Christian healing in the public domain because of Lake's own accredited medical basis (Lyall 1995). Within the approach I take, in which material from public policy and mental health history are viewed, bridging allows passage between the substance of advocacy and the overarching normative discipline of Practical Theology. In turn, this formally situates advocacy in a theological framework because of the spiritual origins of Clinical Theology. In addition, since advocacy as a professional and statutory practice is relatively new in the UK, it will give greater purchase to the impact of Practical Theology in the public sphere because of the harmonisation of the many sources within the argument.[5]

Further to the definitional discussion, Stephen Pattison, Professor of Religion, Ethics and Practice at the University of Birmingham, and a senior figure in the area (Bennett 2012, p. 481), called for extensive use of the theory, empiricism, insights and methods of the social sciences belonging to the discipline. Along with Ballard (2000), Pattison (2007b) noted that Practical Theology was not an esoteric practice which could be ignored by non-theologians since he found that it was shaped by notions of interdisciplinarity, 'humanisation,' social usefulness, welfare and health promotion (S. Pattison 2007b, p. 269; see also S. Pattison 1994). As I acknowledge, advocacy is often considered a wholly secular, and not a theological, endeavour in itself, but since it exists in the health and social care domain, the social welfare reach of Practical Theology can encompass independent advocacy. Broad social science is drawn on to inform analysis and provide that bridge into a practical theological disciplinary arena wherein I marshal evidence, the implications of which radiate back out into the health and social care environment.

Pattison (2000) regretted that 'pastoral care' had 'depressingly' contributed little to wider debates about care and well-being in secular society and imports from other disciplines rather than exporting to them (S. Pattison 2000, p. 205). This book reverses that trend by the outstanding social feature of independent advocacy and linking it with Practical

---

[5] In Lake's 'Dynamic Cycle,' acceptance preceded achievement with the need to identify with the sufferer (patient) and to subjugate one's personal agenda to that of the other. The Hebrew Bible was referenced: 'Then I came to them of the captivity at Tel-Aviv, and I sat where they sat and remained there astonished' (Ezekiel 3:10–15, Bible). This motif is taken up below in relation to advocacy (see, for example, http://www.bridgepastoral.org.uk/dynamic-cycle.htm).

Theology, by, on the one hand, beginning a conversation on how reflection on the spirituality latent in advocacy could affect its theoretical status and, on the other hand, by discussing approaches to advocacy within spiritual practices, such as hospital chaplaincy.

Pattison (2000) wrote that there is 'no reason at all why practical theology... should not extend its influence beyond the confines of the Christian community to consider other issues, e.g. those with mental health problems' (S. Pattison 2000, p. 205). And Pattison has himself also contributed to the debate about professionalisation. Conscious that Practical Theology is a relatively new development within an ancient discipline, to paraphrase Swinton (Swinton and Mowat 2006, p. 7), advocacy practice will, I argue, be seen to have a *telos* (or purpose) to improve human experience and expectation. The literature and the Care Act 2014 show how commissioning factors have heralded the introduction of more formal recognition, for example, the Independent Advocacy qualification (IAQ) and related debates about professionalisation have brought a rigour to a discipline marked by adaptability to individuals being supported in that field.

In summary, there are important historical streams behind the development of Practical Theology in the situation of advocacy. There has not been space here to discuss these in detail above, but other narratives show how the history of pastoral care, counselling and psychotherapy, influenced by advances in the USA, fostered a relationship between theology and pastoral care which has found increased social and political contextualisation in the UK. This also emerged with a formal place for Practical Theology in the academic theological community both in curricula and journals. For example, the pastoral/practical theologian Alastair Campbell had a role at one point in resisting an American clericalised model of clinical pastoral education (CPE) by publishing a paper by Robert Lambourne in the journal *Contact* in 1971 (Lyall 2010).[6]

---

[6] Alongside this account, there was a balancing concern, according to chaplain and researcher Copsey (2012), that spiritual care (or the Practical Theology associated with this occupation) was yet to establish an evidence base. This factor is important because of the way in which I pair the occupation of chaplain with that of the advocate. More positive in his assessment of US influence in the sector, Copsey (2012) thought that while psychology had been seen as a peripheral discipline in mental health in the UK in 1985, it proceeded from that time to evidence outcomes with a more comprehensive research base, as it already did in the USA. It was therefore for chaplaincy to emu-

Having set advocacy practice and theory in the creative and public disciplinary area of Practical Theology, I now move on to the means by which findings in this work were generated and interpreted in accordance with the worldview I espouse. The literature I draw on has a key role in outlining how I am establishing principles and features of the argument which carries the story.

The literature and examples I select provide a background narrative drawn from aspects of spiritual history, scriptures and tradition in order to interrogate the emerging philosophical basis of advocacy as it grew out of mental health history and acquired a separate status (MacDonald 2007; K. Newbigging et al. 2015; K. a. Newbigging and McKeown 2007; Pesut 2008; Sellman 2000). Within the discipline of Practical Theology, a critical conversation will occur between independent advocacy and both spirituality and theology so that different sources are excavated using cases (M. Brown 2007). There certainly is little literature in the UK which I have been able to find which has attempted specifically to develop a theology of advocacy; one exception may be Gammack (2011a). I will draw on his 'liberational' vision of advocacy (Gammack 2011a, b). Considerable work, however, has been done in the area of relating spirituality with mental health (Gilbert 2011; Reinders 2008; Royal-College-of-Psychiatrists'-Spirituality-and-Psychiatry-Special-Interest-Group-Executive-Committee 2010).

3   Personal Introduction

I was employed as a full-time IMCA in the voluntary sector (2005–2011) and later as a hospital chaplain (from 2011), both in London, England. This vantage point seemed to offer an unusual mix of experiences which

---

late that process. Associated with this was the fact that counselling psychology also had a ready-made research base in the USA, which was imported into the UK. However, research and activity at the Cardiff Centre for Chaplaincy Studies (Cardiff University), the Oxford Centre for Ecclesiology and Practical Theology (Oxcept) and the British and Irish Association for Practical Theology (BIAPT)—which had produced the journal, *Contact*, renamed *Practical Theology*—began to meet the need for evidence-based studies, and to generate an indigenously British Practical Theology appropriate for the chaplaincy sector and, by extension, the welfare-based health economy in the UK (Copsey 1997, 2012). My text should be seen partly as a response to Copsey's (2012) challenge to produce a research base.

enriched each other. Previously a teacher, during my ministerial training in England I became interested in Practical Theology (which, as noted above, incorporates the social and psychological dimensions of pastoral practice). Although I may be challenged for taking a broadly Christian perspective, this angle is justified and balanced by my experience in diverse health and social care and in multi-faith service management from 2005 and since most participating advocates, whom I highlight, did not subscribe to any faith position.

From this viewpoint I could make close observations. In his work Mason (2002) pinpointed the 'discipline of noticing' and made the link between reflective and professional practice, and research. The particular point I make evolved from trends and issues to do with professionalisation, which I had noticed within the advocacy sector. For this evolving 'reflective practitioner,' it helped to be ordained in the Church of England (as I was in 1991) and my early research interest grew out of cross-cultural studies at Masters' level. For this I had interviewed theological teachers and students about social and cultural aspects of change (Morgan 1997). Further social interest was broadened and consolidated when I was a Patient and Public Involvement Forum (PPIF)[7] coordinator with various London National Health Service (NHS) trusts (2005–2007). Following this, I received statutory training as an IMCA and also worked as Professional (instructed) Advocate with a number of London boroughs (local authorities) (2007–2011). These areas have been subject to the trade winds of change on the seas of the UK NHS and social care movements I wished to chart. In addition, since my employment as a healthcare chaplain from July 2011, I found that the new professional perspective assisted in accounting for my experience in advocacy.

The primary field to which I went for interviews was that of advocacy. I also interviewed those outside that field in order to gain other perspectives on advocacy skills and experience. Based on concepts developed in the fieldwork period, I interviewed employees and clients of voluntary organisations, and spiritual care coordinators/chaplains for the project.

---

[7] PPIFs were set up as statutory bodies under the now defunct Commission for Patient and Public Involvement in Health. This became Local Involvement Networks (LINkS) in 2008, and then (Local) Healthwatch (2012) and related to local authorities rather than healthcare trusts in order to strengthen local accountability. I discuss this history and further transformations of this body below.

The results of these interviews, transcribed and analysed, are the basis for the narrative which I set out. The participants, whose details and organisational affiliations are anonymised, are listed in Appendix 2 along with a few questionnaire recipients. They were advocates employed by or volunteering with independent advocacy organisations in the London area that received no direct funding from the NHS and clients of advocacy organisations who had experienced or experience mental disorders, *or* mild learning disabilities, but were not subject to the Mental Capacity Act (MCA) 2005. They also included NHS-funded chaplains. Of these there was a balance of male and female participants and a spread between those over and under the age of 40. More precise quantitative-type analysis, for example, regarding age, gender and ethnicity, although important, was not deliberately included in the sourcing of participants, but diverse cultural and spiritual backgrounds were definitely crucial in producing relevant findings. See Table 1.1

4   Perspectives on Professionalisation

In her study of professionalism comparing the fields of medicine, the law and the clergy, the ethicist, Daryl Koehn (1994) argued that an academic description of professionalism should not ignore the nature of that profession and its relationship to other human activities. In this present work I want to consider expressions of the occupation of 'independent advocate,' described briefly here as a specific social care role which supports less able individuals with life choices, as it evolved and became statutory. In order to put the account into perspective I will explore what (as indicated at the outset) at first sight is a basic human activity, which at some given point any of us may formally require in the same way as we may need, for example, medical treatment. Koehn maintained that the sum total of 'what professionals actually did' could not alone constitute a norm for that profession (Koehn 1994, pp. 6–7). That is why I will view a range of activities under the heading of advocacy in order to construct an account of this emergent professional identity and to understand the impact in other areas, such as the social and spiritual formation of indi-

Table 1.1 Fieldwork activity

Given name(s) of participant n = 40	Date of interview (Q denotes questionnaire only)	Category	Numbered lines	Data source by code (location and status)
Angela	1-10-2007	Advocate	202	B2/A1
Bernard	19-8-2008	Chaplain	336	T1/C1
Dorothy	18-9-2008	Chaplain	291	T2/C2
Fauzia	1-10-2007	Advocate	130	B1/A2
Jana	22-10-2007	Advocate	130	B6/A3
Janine	1-10-2007	Advocate	199	B3/A4
Karim and Sarah	4-12-2008	Chaplains	369	N2/C3&4
Kevin	14-1-2008	Advocate	275	BB1/A5
Louise, Michael, Pixy, Whitney and Germaine (n = 5)	23-11-2007	Clients/ self- advocates	205	U1/SA1-5
Maria	1-10-2007	Advocate	122	B4/A6
Micky, Einstein, Yolanda, Norma, Robert, Madonna, Scooby and Barry (n = 8)	14-5-2008	Clients/ self- advocates	210	BB2/SA6-13)
Nigel and Colin	11-9-2008	Chaplains	295	TT1/C4&5
Norah and Bella	14-12-2009	Advocates	806	BB4/A7&8
Nebi	22-10-2007	Advocate	150	B5/A9
Olive	7-11-2007	Advocate	207	U2/A10
Peter	9-12-2008	Advocate	272	BB5/A11
Ruth	21-11-2007	Advocate	202	Z/A12
Sam	13-2-2008	Advocate	236	BB3/A13
Zablon	19-9-2008	Chaplain	226	TT2/C6
TX	(Q) 5-2008	Advocate		Q1/A14
HX	(Q) 7-2008	Advocate		Q2/A15
IK	(Q) 6-2008	Advocate		Q3/A16
JJ	(Q) 4-2008	Advocate		Q4/A17
SS	(Q) 7-2008	Advocate		Q5/A18
CE	(Q) 12-2008	Board member		Q6/D1
LL	(Q) 8-2008	Advocate		Q7/A19

viduals involved in the practice. I will see how these related forces can be given shape to produce more culturally and spiritually attuned norms, seeking a refreshed model of advocacy.

As to consideration of whether the advocate's place of work is worthy of research, Eraut (2004) spoke of the 'under-researched... workplace' and community contexts; he indicated new perspectives encompassing less structured environments and classified 'informal learning' as providing greater flexibility and opportunities to benefit from 'learning that takes place in the spaces surrounding activities and events' (Eraut 2004, p. 247).[8] This book is founded upon sustained human and spiritual reflection on my knowledge and experience in a certain developing workplace, namely advocacy schemes in the voluntary and community sector, and over a limited period (2005–2012), and is intended to enlarge a small, almost negligible, body of formally researched knowledge. Further to this orientation via professional studies, the discipline of Practical Theology was for Pattison (2007a) a focus for the interrogation of human sciences and for research to emerge from pastoral practice (S. Pattison 2007a). In common with advocacy, Practical Theology needed, according to Miller-McLemore (2012) 'succinct and expansive' definitions so that theology could impact upon public life.

5   'Speaking up for Others'

In inviting the reader to consider the definitions of advocacy in more detail, I sense that these reveal aspects of the likely future of social care in which the range of options from patient to friend, carer and volunteer or paid advocate are more depended upon within the constraints of the health economy. The discrete area of 'patient advocacy,' commonly used in American literature, became a subject line in the International Nursing Index in 1976. Within the UK, articles following the US trend reached high points in the early-1980s and the mid-1990s (numbering 100 US

---

[8] In terms of informal learning, Jarvis (1999) stated that a body of researched knowledge is crucial for 'occupations that are professionalising' and that 'practitioners produce their own personal theory as a result of reflecting on their own work' (Jarvis 1999, pp. 36, 149).

and 50 UK), with a low of 10–30 articles in the late 1980s (Mallik and Rafferty 2000). The definition of the independent (rather than the legal) advocate is an individual who supports another with capacity or mental health problems in decision-making. This spans the fields of health and social care both in the USA and the UK, but in this book I consider only London, UK. Emerging from US consumer rights movements of the 1970s, the existence of 'patients' rights advocates' begged the question of whether it was a role which should be performed by nurses (Bateman 2000; Llewellyn and Northway 2007; Ravich and Schmolka 1996). What prevents social workers and other practitioners 'advocating' for their clients? (Mallik 1998). Mallik (1997) thought advocacy a 'risky role to adopt' for nurses and later found that the rejection by the nursing elite of the professionalisation of the role of nurse-advocate opened up a gap (Mallik 1997, p. 130). This gap could be occupied by independent advocacy because it was separated by definition from 'the system.'

Atkinson, an authority often cited, defined it as 'speaking up' because, as mentioned initially, 'everyone, sooner or later, needs help in making their voice heard – and advocates are people who can provide the time and support to enable this to happen' (Atkinson 1999, pp. 5–9; Henderson 2005, p. 206). The 'time and support to enable voices to be heard' happens in a variety of forms, further delineated below. I see this definition has an historical grounding, which I deal with later, but firstly let us view the range of current practices.

5.1   Instructed or Non-instructed Advocacy?

Firstly, activities which support those who can request, or direct, that support in order to be able to 'speak up' for themselves and who can exercise choices count as 'instructed advocacy,' which includes mental health advocacy and the statutory role of the Independent Mental Health Advocate (IMHA). By contrast, 'non-instructed advocacy' focuses on more disabled or vulnerable individuals who have been deemed to lack specific capacity and therefore need specialist support in 'best interests' decisions. The occupation as a whole, therefore, exists to ensure that principles of choice, equality and justice are observed in relation to information exchange, making a complaint or taking decisions. These concerns usually relate to the health and social care system (e.g. mental health or learning disabilities), employment or housing, but may also include safeguarding (vulnerable) adults or children (formerly adult or child protection). The form of advocacy which is accordingly required will depend on the client group.

The subsequent element in this definition—concerning principles— was strengthened by statute in 2007 to formally represent the wishes and preferences, beliefs and values of a client—for example, in the IMCA non-instructed advocacy role when a client lacks capacity to make a specific decision or in the IMHA role where the individual referred has capacity to give an instruction regarding their support.

> The statutory principles aim to: protect people who lack capacity and help them take part, as much as possible, in decisions that affect them. They aim to assist and support people who may lack capacity to make particular decisions, not to restrict or control their lives. (Chancellor 2007, p. 20)

This IMCA role was also extended through the Deprivation of Liberty Safeguards (DoLS) legislation (6.3.3.). From April 2009, safeguards were implemented further designed to protect the interests of a mentally vulnerable group of service-users (those sectioned in mental health units) to ensure they were given the care they needed in 'less restrictive' regimes and to prevent arbitrary decisions which deprived them of their liberty (DoH 2008b; Pritchard 2009, p. 144ff). This statutory role came in alongside the more traditional non-statutory advocacy role, which supports clients with decision-making capacity to speak up about wishes and beliefs, and to ensure that their voices are heard and actions taken to extend rights and choices. I will relate this activity further below to spiritual motivations via the Practical Theology perspective.

5.2   Differing Forms of Independent Advocacy

Extensive roots in advocacy have led to a diversity of expressions in practice, including, firstly, 'citizen advocacy,' which involves volunteers recruited, supported and trained by a coordinator who matches them with people who are not well able to defend their rights as citizens. The work is 'one-to-one,' can last a long time and usually applies in relation to people with learning disabilities. Secondly, 'peer advocacy' applies when the advocate has something in common with the person they are advocating for—for example, they may be a user or ex-user of services. Importantly, both of these forms count as volunteer advocacy: this would involve volunteers working alongside paid advocates, holding a small caseload and offering support to individuals. Thirdly, 'group or collective advocacy' happens when individuals come together for a particular issue, but it may need independent facilitation of resources. Fourthly, 'self-advocacy,' the most empowering form of the practice, encompasses the idea of individuals speaking up for themselves. All modes of advocacy would aim to promote self-advocacy in their design, and it would be the ideal to aim towards, according to the ethos of advocacy. Finally, 'professional, paid or specialist advocacy' (as in IMCA and IMHA) usually involves casework and adopts a problem-solving approach in relation to the outcome desired by the client being supported, or the decision-maker if the client is not able to instruct the advocate. The advocate may be trained, engaged in professional development or have developed specific knowledge of systems and services, and support the person through them (Henderson 2005, p. 205; Henderson and Pochin 2001).

Henderson (2005) described advocacy by defining what it is not: it is not advice, befriending, mediation, counselling or social work, according to the writer. But it is about choice, social inclusion, equality, justice, support, empowerment, protection and information (Henderson 2005, p. 205). This assumes the independence of the advocate. If the 'central tenet of independence is missing from an advocacy relationship in which the advocate is also acting as a professional…' (Forbat and Atkinson 2005, p. 331), a statement which reveals the shortcomings of the role applied sometimes to the nurse or social worker, recent developments have reasserted the inherent desirability of independence in advocacy practice. The deployment of advocates in the introduction of the state-funded statutory Independent Complaints and Advocacy Service (ICAS) in September 2003 (Dimond 2003), IMCA services in April 2007 (Gorczynska 2007) provided by voluntary organisations and the IMHA and IMCA DoLS in 2009 were evidence of strategic planning for the independent role (see further below c (iv)).

In summary, independent advocacy consists of a service staffed by volunteers or professionals from a voluntary or non-profit organisation, commissioned by a local authority or primary care trust in which practitioners support individuals to make choices, take decisions and secure rights in relation to health, social care and housing; this activity may take place on an instructed or non-instructed basis if individuals lack capacity to make certain decisions. Having reached a definition of independent advocacy, for initial clarity of focus I will present a snapshot of the status quo regarding statutory advocacy in England and Wales in the last ten years, followed by the narrative of the broader historical and theological lead-in, as I have observed it.

6   Advocacy and Public Policy

6.1   Statutory Advocacy, User Focus, and English Public Policy 2005–2015

The year 2007 was a ground-breaking year in the development of professional advocacy as a prominent feature in the health and social care landscape in the UK (England and Wales) in that, firstly, the MCA 2005 came into force on April 1, with the publication of a Code of Practice, and with other provisions of the Act coming into force on October 1 of that year.

> The Act requires a range of people to 'have regard' to the Code, for example those acting in relation to a person lacking capacity in a paid or professional role. On 1 April 2007, those aspects of the Act relating to Independent Mental Capacity Advocates and the new criminal offence of ill-treatment or neglect came into force. (Ministerial-Statement 2007)

And, secondly, the Mental Health Act (MHA) 1983 was revised (and implemented in 2009), which led to a statutory IMHA service and created a duty 'to provide advocacy services for all detained patients…, guardianship patients and patients subject to community treatment orders.'

There was a new duty upon service providers to provide qualifying patients with information that advocacy services were available, an unfettered right to meet with patients in private and to meet with professionals. Advocates were also given access to patient records but 'only where a capable patient gives consent, or, in the case of an incapable patient, where such access would not conflict with a decision made by a deputy, donee, court etc., and the person holding the records agrees that such access is "appropriate"' (Mental-Health-Act-Commission 2007).

This had been in place since April 2009 with the Code of Practice having been consulted upon and some training given. Furthermore, these changes had been formalised after a period of years in gestation due to social and political pressures. In April 2007 the Department of Health facilitated the commissioning of IMCA services nationally through voluntary organisations in each borough in England. The MHA had been under parliamentary scrutiny for over 25 years since its first introduction in 1983. The MCA was introduced originally as the 'Mental Incapacity Bill' in 2003. A greater respect for patients' views, an espousal of holistic rather than medical models alone, was indicated. For Gilbert (2007b), the NHS Care and Community Act (1990) had made it a duty for local authorities to assess people for social care and support so that 'people who "appear to need community care services" are entitled to an assessment – (and) the results of the assessment will determine whether services should be provided…' (Gilbert 2007b).

Bowl (1996) had detailed the legislation for user involvement and was rather pessimistic about its real effect (Bowl 1996), but Gilbert (2007b) stated that its increase in the last 15 years, as we have noted above (Atkinson 1999, p. 9; Pilgrim and Waldron 1998), was among the reasons for the changes in the system:

> The launch of the Government's Social Inclusion Report on Mental Health in the summer of 2004, has raised the profile of the need for organisations to consider their Whole Persons' and Whole Systems' Approaches. (Gilbert 2007b)

The Adult Care White Paper 'Our Health, Our Care, Our Say' (DH 2006) and the 'DH Commissioning Guidance' (2007) put forward a personalised approach to care based on user choice and control. The link with user involvement was identified by Bradshaw (2008), who was optimistic that 'involvement policies (which) began as benign benevolence' had turned users into 'the means to distributing resources in a way that was originally unintended' as far as personalisation was concerned (P.L. Bradshaw 2008). Gilbert continued to point out that the Commission on Integration and Cohesion, in its report 'Our Shared Future' (2007), also made proposals for social cohesion, 'which must include faith communities' (Gilbert 2007a). This often applied to individuals with learning disabilities.[9]

According to Ramcharan and Grant writing in 2001, 'people with learning disabilities... have little control over their own lives, though almost all, including the most severely disabled, are capable of making choices and expressing their views and preferences' (DoH 2001, para. 4.1, p. 44). These were the functions in which professional advocates would involve themselves. Campbell, a 'service recipient' himself, wrote that the quality of a service-user's involvement and the effectiveness in services 'may be improved if they have access to an independent advocate' (Campbell 2001, p. 87). It was even more important to establish the views of those who found it hard to participate actively (DoH 1990, para. 3.16, p. 25) and to establish partnerships (NHS Executive 1996), they stated (Ramcharan and Grant 2001). Relative to this, the role of the

---

[9] The emphasis on 'personalisation' thus gained in intensity in 2007 and 2008 (Hampshire-County-Council 2008; Peter Scourfield 2008) and in Department of Health documents ((DoH) 2007, 2008c, 2008d), and the importance of culture, spirituality and/or faith had been rising also. Both of these tendencies can be linked to the growth of the user movement in the previous 15 years (Atkinson 1999, p. 9; Pilgrim and Waldron 1998). Little has been done to reflect theologically upon these changes although the social value (or capital) in faith has been re-emphasised (Furbey and Joseph Rowntree 2006). Ramcharan and Grant (2001) underlined the point about rising user choice and control in the light of the discussion above, and regarding patient and public involvement (PPI) and user involvement:

> In the areas of policy and practice guidance, the past decade has witnessed an unprecedented growth in calls for the involvement and participation of users. Much policy has repeated the view that 'most people can express their own views if we are prepared to get to know them, to understand them and to respond to them' (NHS Executive 1998, para. 2.2, p. 3; see also DoH 1998a), (Ramcharan and Grant 2001)

IMCA—for a smaller number of people—was precisely to establish the views, preferences, beliefs and values of individuals who cannot actively participate at all in a decision needing to be made, as indeed the role of the spiritual care coordinator/chaplain might be to ensure that spiritual assessments take place and that these forms of needs are met. I will deal with some issues below (6.3.4.) which are raised by means of an examination of advocacy training initiatives which have become mandatory for advocacy schemes, and in Chap. 6 I will consider how Practical Theology could enhance these. Having discussed how an advocate may assist with the provision of services, I will now show how advocacy has entered the public arena in terms of policy development in the formation of recent health and social care policy.

6.2   Advocacy Discussed in the British Parliament

Following the launch of debates on the Health and Social Care Bill from February 2011 onwards, on 16 May, 2011, a Member of the House of Commons tabled eight questions on advocacy. The Secretary of State for Health was asked what steps he was taking to ensure that local advocacy services meet the needs of people with profound and multiple learning disabilities, about the monitoring and assessing of those services, about skills and training development for advocates, about individual care packages, about safeguarding the interests of these people, and regarding costs. The then Minister, Paul Burstow, responded that it was up to 'local authorities to decide how much advocacy they commission for people with profound and multiple learning disabilities, who they commission it from and how they make it available to their local populations.' The role of the Department is to provide the framework for services—to be clear about social care law and about social care policy, the Minister stated. Therefore, he said, the Government was considering the report of the Law Commission and looking to modernise the legal framework in which social care was provided (Commons 2011).

He mentioned the influence of the then proposed legislation and stated that 'subject to the passage of the Health and Social Care Bill, local authorities and general practitioner commissioning consortia will be required to prepare a Joint Strategic Needs Assessment (JSNA).' The bill underwent amendments and was enacted in March 2012 with significant references to advocacy (Section 185). So, according to Burstow, the Act was intended to ensure that each area developed a comprehensive analysis of their current and future needs (including those relevant to health, social care and public health), which was where advocacy providers were affected. Based on the JSNA, the members of the committees were required to develop a joint health and well-being strategy for their area, according to Burstow (Commons 2011).

To further explore the minister's concerns about advocacy, he had referred to the Government document *Vision for Adult Social Care, Capable Communities and Active Citizens*, which argued that 'councils should focus on improving the range, quality and accessibility of information, advice and advocacy available for all people in their communities—regardless of how their care is paid for—to support their social care choices' (Dept.-of-Health 2010a). In answering the questions, Burstow also singled out IMCA and the £6 million made available to local authorities to commission local services to provide for the IMCA role. Drawing on the 2010 IMCA Annual Report (Dept-of-Health 2010b), he said that 10,000 people benefited from this in 2010. Focusing on training, Burstow referred to Department of Health support for advocacy training:

> The Department has worked with the advocacy sector to develop a national qualification in advocacy, which is available to the sector and to commissioners. The national advocacy qualification has been part of the professionalising of advocacy and ensures that advocates are appropriately trained. The Department has also funded a 'Quality Mark' system, administered by Action for Advocacy, which enable advocacy organisations to demonstrate their services are of high quality. (Commons 2011)

He added that 'the Department does not collect local information on advocacy provision and its costs,' a statement which emphasised the importance of the relationship of the local advocacy provider with the commissioners.

It may be interesting to note that many of my concerns as author, which I raised at the outset—in particular, the question dealt with in this book regarding the relationship between professionalisation and practice in advocacy—were reiterated in these questions in Parliament in May 2011, when the impact of NHS financial cuts plus the introduction of the social care bill and subsequent Health and Social Care Act made themselves felt, as will be noted further below.

6.3   Statutory Independent Advocacy: 2011 to the Present

6.3.1   NHS Complaints Advocacy

The Health and Social Care Act 2012 seriously impacted the expansion of advocacy services in this period. The introduction of a right to support in making complaints, similar to the service which the ICAS, begun in 2003, and later the Citizens' Advice Bureaux provided, was pushed out more widely to advocacy providers, either directly, or through Healthwatch, the public watchdog successor to LINkS (Local Involvement Networks). This was enacted from April 2013 (in section 185, mentioned above), and, in turn, an amendment to section 223 of the Local Government and Public Involvement in Health Act 2007 (Legislation.gov.uk 2012). The word on 'advocacy street' is that the inclusion of complaints has significantly increased the workload for advocacy providers; the service is advertised on websites as free independent support, not advice, but open nonetheless to all who may wish to complain (Personal communication 2015).

6.3.2   Post-legislative Scrutiny of the Mental Health Act 2013 and Care Act 2014

In 2013 the Response to the Report of the Commons Health Committee to Post-Legislative Scrutiny of the MHA 2007 recommended as the fourth of its 12 recommendations that the IMHA service become 'opt-out' rather than 'opt-in,' which would have a significant effect on the remit of mental health advocates. This was impacted by the respected

University of Central Lancashire's 2012 report (Department-of-Health 2013; Newbigging et al. 2012).

Elsewhere, the health and social care legislation was finalised in 2014, known as the 'Care Act.' Sections 67 and 68 drew advocacy provision further in by placing a duty on local authorities from April 2015 to make sure that information and advice on care and support were also available. It stated that independent advocacy must be arranged if a person would otherwise 'be unable to participate in, or understand, the care and support system' (The-College-of-Social-Work/Skills-for-Care 2014).

The Act effectively underlined principles of the MCA 2005 and clearly supported the statutory option of involving an independent advocate in safeguarding adults cases. The key phrase was 'substantial difficulty,' as can be seen from this excerpt:

'See for section 67 (4)

4. The condition is that the local authority considers that, were an independent advocate not to be available, the individual would experience *substantial difficulty* in doing one or more of the following— (my italics)

(a) understanding relevant information;

(b) retaining that information;

(c) using or weighing that information as part of the process of being involved;

(d) communicating the individual's views, wishes or feelings (whether by talking, using sign language or any other means).' (Legislation.gov.uk 2014)

The subsequent increase in Care Review referrals has had a comprehensive impact on advocacy services; additionally I have heard of a London borough which makes a safeguarding referral conditional upon availability of an advocate, so the overall message is that this has had an overwhelming effect on these services (Personal communication 2015).

6.3.3   Deprivation of Liberty Safeguards and Cheshire West

Two other events in 2014 have had an effect on IMCAs and on advocacy generally. On 13 March, a House of Lords Select Committee found that the DoLS were not fit for purpose, but were overly complex and bureaucratic. A few days later, on 19 March, Lady Hale pronounced judgement in the 'Cheshire West' Case in the UK Supreme Court, that two individuals with learning disabilities in that borough, despite appearances to the contrary, were, in fact, deprived of their liberty. This would unexpectedly put pressure on social services (including, quite possibly, IMCA) because it meant that anyone experiencing constant 'control and supervision' could be subject to a DoLS. Precisely, the UK Supreme Court clarified the 'acid test' of deprivation of liberty as constituting whether an individual 'lacks the mental capacity to consent to the arrangements for their care **and** is under continuous control and supervision **and** is not free to leave their place of residence' (Department-of-Health 2014, p. 32).

The result of both these outcomes, including a government response, was an increase in DoLS referrals in health and social care. This made an impression in the arena of NHS acute intensive care services in that it was said that theoretically anyone lacking capacity due to an injury should be referred, and a tenfold increase in referrals resulted and more temporary authorisations than could be dealt with (Commons 2014; Department-of-Health 2014, p. 32).

6.3.4   Advocacy Training

Finally, in the Seventh Annual IMCA Service Report (2013–2014), the theme of training arose again, with a baseline minimum training required via in-service training (based on a Lords' recommendation), with a comprehensive framework of six capabilities. This was enunciated in Appendix D:

Key capability 1:   The ability to have a sound understanding of, and keep up-to-date with, the MCA, DoLS and other relevant legislative frameworks and relevant case law

Key capability 2:   The ability to work in a manner that promotes the MCA and the rights of those who may be affected by the MCA

Key capability 3:   The ability to have a sound understanding of capacity assessments, best practice and creative assessments and the ability to challenge capacity assessments in an

Key capability 4:   appropriate and outcome focused manner when relevant to do so

Key capability 4:   The ability to promote supported decision making for those who lack capacity: i.e. ensuring decisions made on behalf of those who lack capacity start from the point of view of the person and not the opinions of those in control of making those decisions

Key capability 5:   The ability to deliver high quality instructed and non-instructed advocacy when carrying out the IMCA roles: namely: a. Change of accommodation b. Serious medical treatment c. Care reviews d. Adult protection e. s.39A f. s.39C g. s.39D

Key capability 6:   Additional safeguard i.e. challenging decisions formally and informally (Department-of-Health 2014, p. 46)

To put this in context, I consider briefly some moves in the prior development of training. In recent history, from January 2007 a training manager was appointed to research and further develop the suite of qualifications arising from the initial IMCA training material. The generic advocacy qualification had four modules which together entitled the completing learner to a Level 3 Advocacy Qualification. The suite included training for IMHAs and children's advocates amongst five specialist four-day courses which led to Level 4 advocacy qualifications. The IMCA units became modules in the subsequent IMCA qualification, and the training started in January 2009 (D. Barnes 2006; Department-of-Health-and-the-Welsh-Assembly 2008).

The new qualification was based on a Vocational Related Qualification (VRQ) model, rather than a National Vocational Qualification (NVQ), and was validated by City and Guilds: 'VRQs are qualifications that concentrate on the knowledge relating to a specific vocational area, e.g. Learning Disability. NVQs are qualifications that concentrate on the skills and competence relating to a general vocational area, e.g. Care.' ((DoH) and The-British-Institute-of-Human-Rights 2007). It was based on the National Occupational Standards and consisted of ten taught days. IMCAs, who had previously undergone the initial course, were required to present a portfolio of their practice in order to be awarded the formal qualification.

Kate Mercer, the national training manager (at the time) summarised the problem, which had been uncovered in a consultation process she had engaged in with advocacy service providers and organisations in relation to the proposed NAQ/IAQ. Some of those surveyed saw advocacy as a service for which professionalism and accountability would bring an improvement in services which were provided. Others, contrarily, saw the very same scenario as a threat because they viewed advocacy as a movement with few, if any, boundaries (Mercer 2007).

Elsewhere and earlier, a number of advocates and advocacy organisations had expressed serious reservations about the concept and nature of training for advocates.

> Within citizen advocacy schemes, the concept of 'advocate training' is anathema in that citizen advocates are ordinary people who bring their own skills, knowledge and experiences to the advocacy relationship. Many citizen advocacy schemes do not even use the term 'training' to describe the support offered to advocates, preferring 'orientation.' (Henderson and Pochin 2001, p. 149)

Also, in 2005 advocates were interviewed on their experience in mental health settings; they then 'felt under-trained but training was seen as essential in ensuring some standardization of practice, reassuring health care practitioners of the legitimacy of the advocates' role,' and that it would help to bring in funding and give volunteer advocates a 'career pathway' (Carver and Morrison 2005, p. 77).

Furthermore, an Action for Advocacy[10] discussion forum elicited the following contributions:

> I would quite like to become an excellent advocate and I would quite like a certificate that says I have done the training... Does having a qualification necessarily mean professionalism is the end result? Could the training actually include how 'not' to be 'professional'? (Henderson 2007, p. 17)

It was also feared among smaller advocacy organisations that the introduction of a NAQ/IAQ would result in a two-tier system with those from larger organisations better able to afford to pay for the training of

---

[10] A fine support and training broker for advocates, which went unfunded.

advocates, thus sending unqualified advocates to the bottom of the pile. In addition, should commissioners make the NAQ a condition of obtaining funding, then smaller schemes would be edged out of the advocacy market. Henderson commented that if it is 'too costly, time-consuming or academic then it will alienate smaller schemes and volunteers, who are such an integral part of a diverse sector' (Henderson 2007, p. 17).

All things considered, seven years later and in the Commons response to the Lord's Select Committee report, the government's commitment to and enthusiasm for the MCA and advocates as 'of fundamental importance' was very heartening. It pointed to the MCA and advocacy as a means to address failings at Winterbourne View and Mid-Staffordshire NHS Foundation Trust, linking it with the documents *Transforming Care* (the national response to Winterbourne View) and *Hard Truths* (the government response to the *Francis Report* into the failings at Mid-Staffordshire).

> The MCA is also a key contributor to achieving the aims of the Equality Act 2010 and the United Nations Convention on the Rights of Persons with Disabilities through its principle of treating all individuals equally and without discrimination (Commons 2014, p. 9).

For these reasons I am proud to be associated with advocacy's passage into the mainstream and redouble my concern to explore its spiritual dimensions, which are hinted at in the baseline minimum requirements in 2 (a) as 'understanding the impact of cultural, religious and social differences' (Department-of-Health 2014, p. 42).

7   The Argument in Brief

My argument relates to issues about the development of advocacy as a professionalised occupation in England and Wales from 2005 onwards. As the statutory requirement for IMCAs and IMHAs passed into English and Welsh law in 2007 and 2009, respectively, I considered that this highlighted the growing significance of advocacy in health and social care and the emergence of these particular roles as occupations undergoing professionalisation. I view social policy changes, the advancing consciousness of human rights, and broader awareness of cultural and spiritual influences occurring in the same areas as evidence of the above.

My purpose is to explain how these social and cultural pressures affect the evolution of advocacy as an occupation as it is shaped into a profession. Independent advocacy has its roots in altruistic and spiritual soil, and specifically in its European and, to some extent, American expressions within the field of theology. In the next chapters, therefore, advocacy is discerned in early civil, political and human rights movements, mental health history and nursing philosophy. There is also continuity with the voices which herald the arrival of self-conscious advocacy in the twentieth and twenty-first centuries. The increase in the literature of spirituality and mental health, concepts of well-being, empowerment and democratisation in the rising service-user movement are tidal events in identifying a spirituality of advocacy. Compiling a history of independent advocacy with interview material in order to draw out the spiritual, possibly Christian and theological, dimensions is not a task that I am aware has yet been accomplished.

Primarily the role of an advocate, as an independent agent or witness, is distinct from the role which a paid employee of a trust or local authority, such as a nurse or a social worker, could play. Furthermore, the extension of these roles (nurse, social worker) to cover what an independent 'advocate' would, or could do, is rejected. Consequently this leads to an independent 'caring' gap needing to be filled, one which voluntary sector organisations, funded increasingly by central government, can fill. Thus advocacy comes to be separated from 'the system' in order to be better able to support and represent clients, patients or service-users, but in the process it also acquires, in its new-found professionalisation, specific training needs. With the coming of age of advocacy, the question arises whether there is a theoretical paucity in view of what legislative statutes or social workers, consultants or psychiatrists now expect of advocates. Also, because of its spiritual history which I am asserting, approaching advocacy in the framework of Practical Theology enhances its moral and theological basis and can refresh its ethical components.

For the above reasons later I turn to the voluntary and community organisations, the sort I worked within when in the advocacy sector from 2005 to 2011. Empirically the identity of the advocate via the experiences of a number of selected advocacy practitioners and those of their clients reveals new facts which can improve aspects of advocacy practice. The voices of advocates, self-advocates and clients will define normatively the essence of advocacy practice and experience. In addition, conversations are created with voices from another profession—namely, chaplains—within the discipline of Practical Theology, and these are arbitrated by analytical models which apply spiritually and theologically constructed models of empowerment or equal rights—which I shall describe as Reconstructed Empowerment and Action Based on Equality. Based on the interviews, these map respectively the delicate approach advocates adopt to support clients with diminished or no capacity for certain decisions, and the actions taken by them in relation to clients, to rebalance their equality, both legally and spiritually. These themes are interwoven in the text and are expanded on in Chaps. 5 and 6 and in the synthesis of Chap. 7.

The inclusion of chaplains, experienced in pastoral theology in multiple religious traditions, alongside advocates, thus aids deeper excavation into the foundations and implications of independent advocacy in its spiritual (and Christian) rootedness. Both chaplaincy and advocacy are thus linked by this study based in Practical Theology. Parallel to independent advocacy, healthcare chaplaincy is a role which exists to support patients, their relatives and staff but mostly (up to now) on the territory of healthcare trusts in the NHS in England and Wales. Whilst statutory independent advocacy has professional boundaries, there are positive ambiguities with 'voluntary' citizen advocacy, which are mined. Alongside this, existing from the birth of the NHS in 1948, spiritual care exercised in the chaplaincy service in the NHS is a religious and ministerial function which connects with historical faith communities and has a similar semi-independent role in relation to the NHS. The fact that this creative conversation (between advocacy and chaplaincy) will take place within the format of the discipline of Practical Theology may give theological force to my findings.

The history of professionalisation, with which I am concerned in advocacy, also bears similarities with that of chaplaincy.[11] Therefore the merger

---

[11] This includes the political history of the College of Healthcare Chaplains and Multi-Faith Group for Healthcare Chaplaincy (now the 'Healthcare Chaplaincy Faith and Belief Group'), both of

of insights from secular and faith-based advocates, the latter being those who are mostly, but not exclusively, employed as chaplains, takes place to form a particular independent perspective. Independence is important for advocates, and, whilst there is an element of independence in chaplaincy, it is inevitable that chaplains will be employed by NHS trusts and cannot therefore be seen as advocates in the way that advocacy organisations would define the role. The independence of advocates could also be compromised by the fact that, being statutory from 2007, they brought in increasingly boundaried behaviours to which the traditional 'citizen advocate' (mentioned above) was resistant, the sum of which contributes to a profoundly spiritual stance in the ongoing conversation.

It is thus independence within professional advocacy which gives meaning to the activity. Advocacy is commonly understood as a statutory human rights-based expression, much of which is strongly established in UK advocacy legislation.[12] I argue that these policies locate a *conduit* for principles of culture and faith to apply to independent advocacy, underlining why the field of Practical Theology is the best in which to achieve this. How NHS-funded chaplaincy works is not the subject of this book, but similarities with advocacy come from the shared quasi-independent perspective, and it is the basis on which I choose to bring in chaplaincy as a comparator profession, or conversational partner.[13]

---

which used to be part of The Hospital Chaplaincies Council (HCC). In addition, the UK Board of Healthcare Chaplains defines and develops professional standards. The relationships between these bodies have not always been transparent or constructive. Allen (2012).

[12] The statutory responsibility is for those detained under the Mental Health and Capacity Acts to have independent advocacy and for an IMCA advocate, if engaged, to weigh up 'any beliefs and values (e.g. religious, cultural, moral or political) that would be likely to influence the decision in question' (Dept.-for-Constitutional-Affairs 2006b, pp. 20, 65), in accordance with the 'best interests' of a client. Both the Human Rights Act 1998 framework (specifically, Article Nine: Freedom of Conscience [Thought and Religion]) and the fact that public authorities are bound to uphold rights to 'manifest one's religion and beliefs' (Dept.-for-Constitutional-Affairs 2006a) pinpoint the place of faith and spirituality in the process.

[13] National Health Service-funded hospital chaplaincy clearly has a longer and more classical history than advocacy due to the fact that those employed are normally licensed in their own denominations or religions and therefore are carriers of religious heritage. However, there have been threats to the status of chaplaincy since it is not directly related to medical care and can be viewed by some as superfluous in the healthcare environment, especially by secular humanist or atheist critics. The most recent Chaplaincy Guidelines, however, provide space for the spiritual support for those with

Despite its shorter history, could advocacy be in some ways more secure and enduring as a profession than chaplaincy, on account of its human rights and secular basis, and with its comparatively greater level of acceptability due to a gain in status in the last 20 years? Thus the focus of the argument is on advocacy on account of its similar support role to chaplaincy, and where the advocate, like the chaplain, cannot ever be a decision maker. If the role of the advocate contributes to an understanding of chaplaincy, that role could also enhance socially responsible activities in the community and life of the church. This material relates to the second and third of my key questions: how can the practice of advocacy be explained within the framework of the experience of advocacy practitioners, clients and spiritual care professionals or chaplains? and what philosophical or theological models (e.g. Christian ethics, virtue ethics) can be used to consider, better understand and move towards responses to these questions?

Although the expansion of literature in spirituality and mental health is something which some chaplains, or spiritual care coordinators, will be aware of, it represents, especially with some emphasis on generic 'spiritual assessment,' another important angle of which for the advocacy sector to take account. Together I suggest that both mental health chaplaincy and spirituality, mental health theory and some aspects of nursing, which I set out below, are dimensions which benefit from a link with professional advocacy. This connection is broadened and deepened by the exploration of the material from the interview participants.

Against the background of a portrait of the professional activity and reflexivity in the analysis of the interviews with my participants, a culturally and spiritually appropriate model of advocacy based in the discipline of Practical Theology is outlined. By recognising that advocacy appears at first sight to be a thoroughly secular occupation and fulfils a basic humanistic signposting role, voices from advocacy, chaplaincy, nursing philosophy, the relevant literature and public policy are critically correlated to present a theologically informed approach to independent advocacy. Having listened to the voices from all groups, the synthesis-

---

no faith (Swift, Chaplaincy-Leaders-Forum, and National Equality and Health Inequalities Team 2015).

ing practice models of *Reconstructed Empowerment* and *Action Based on Equality* are emblematic of this. The uses (or abuses) of power and equal (or unequal) rights are the substance of advocacy and these 'new' models integrate religious or spiritual elements into advocacy practice within the established remit of Practical Theology. *Spiritual, theological or 'faithful' capital is, I argue, every individual's human right* and is at the heart of independent advocacy. The concepts of Reconstructed Empowerment and Action Based on Equality are related to the third key question, in a new quasi-therapeutic, although resiliently independent, and appropriately culturally and spiritually sensitive space. As well as what spirituality and chaplaincy can bring to advocacy, the question of what independent advocacy may have to say to chaplaincy is raised within the creative and critical conversation. This is why the harmony of the voices of participants is important in order to elucidate these points.

Returning, in conclusion, to the implication of the quotation with which I opened this chapter, skilled paid or voluntary help by another, in the absence of family or friends, is likely to be a necessity for you and me simply to be able to survive. This further example from a textbook on the law and safeguarding (vulnerable) adults pinpointed the advocate's, and the IMCA's role as one that 'cannot be underestimated... (having)

> the scope to have enormous influence for individuals who are unable to state clearly what they want, and are assessed to be unable to make certain decisions. This client group represents some of most vulnerable and potentially disempowered people in society. (Pritchard 2009, p. 151)

Pritchard continued to note how overlooked and marginalised such clients may be: older people with dementia and no family remaining, a young retired person with a brain injury with no known contacts, a younger person with a learning disability whose parents are no longer able to take decisions for her. For these and other people, the resources of advocacy exist and are provided through commissioning arrangements by the state. This would not have been so were it not for a history and the recent activity of advocacy organisations, which, as I will show, have (sometimes subtle) spiritual or theological ramifications of which cognizance must be taken. Christian theology typically and historically characterised such activity, albeit in health and social care, as 'pure religion' in supporting 'widows' and 'orphans' (James 1:27, Bible), while in Islam this is seen as honouring of the principle of Zakat, or charitable giving. As voluntary organisations and their diverse workforce seek to meet increased advocacy needs, broader disciplinary, theoretical and skills bases are required for improved practice. This book seeks to forge paths in this direction.

From this account of the work in progress and in prospect, I will foreground some recent cases before delving into the historical background (Chap. 3) to discern how a 'spiritual vision' of advocacy can highlight how the statutory expressions link with its libertarian and voluntarist heritage and origins. Without recognition of the traditional background, a proposed Practical Theological take on advocacy would be lost. The advent of statutory advocacy has thus had legislative and social force, and social workers, plus more NHS consultants, have at last acquired the word IMCA, as well as IMHA, in their active vocabularies. In the same way that hospitals, for example, grew originally out of monastic foundations with concerns for the poor and diseased, there is a less discerned link between advocacy and its specific spiritual background, which I explore in depth.[14]

---

[14] Bennett (2012) described *The Foundations of Pastoral Studies and Practical Theology* (Ballard 1986) as illustrative of the move in Practical Theology away from 'older models and toward more direct engagement with secular caring and healing professions.' I define Practical Theology as the controlling discipline of this story and where 'more experientially oriented theological reflection on practice' can take place (Bennett 2012, p. 476; Miller-McLemore 2012, pp. 4–5).

2

Selected Case Studies: Independent Mental Capacity Advocacy (IMCA), Mental Health Advocacy, and Deprivation of Liberty Safeguards (DoLS-IMCA)

1   IMCA and Neuro-disabilities

In this chapter there is an initial meeting with some service-users, advocates and spiritual care coordinators via case studies. We consider how some advocates responded to statutory duties under the Mental Capacity Act (MCA) and mental health legislation, and how they support those judged without capacity to be involved in decisions. IMCA is a specialist and non-standard form of advocacy, but on account of its legal and philosophical profile it sharpens thinking in the area. I suggest how spiritual as well as social, cultural, and emotional concerns are included as part of the assessment which the advocate carries out. IMCAs, for example, are bound to produce reports for the decision-maker, which need to be taken account of, before a decision is made.

The information in the two composite case studies below demonstrates some of the concerns which IMCAs and Professional Advocates will bring into the framework of decision-making in relation to those with neuro-disabilities. I will then reflect on the practice based on the following accounts from IMCAs. Names were changed or anonymised, permission

© The Author(s) 2017   **35**
G. Morgan, *Independent Advocacy and Spiritual Care*,
DOI 10.1057/978-1-137-53125-4_2

was sought from the relevant committee and the provider, and details were changed according to the requirements of the MCA. Research can only include 'data that has been anonymised ...' and the 'aim of the research must be to provide knowledge' (about the) 'treatment or care of people with the same impairing condition' (Dept.-for-Constitutional-Affairs. (2006b), pp. 205–7).

1.1   IMCAs and Clients with Acquired Brain Injuries (ABIs)

1.1.1   Case Study 1: Petra

A referral was received from a psychologist regarding Petra's change of accommodation; but there were also safeguarding concerns. The preliminary decision was that on discharge from hospital Petra should move to a nursing service where her needs could be met and also that her friends and family would be able to visit her. Petra was involved in an accident and acquired an injury when on a business trip. She was brought back to the UK for rehabilitation where she was treated in hospitals. Petra was married to an Asian man; she also enjoyed an independent life and was a keen golfer. However, she had a family friend, Betty from the golf club, to whom she had informally entrusted certain decisions (health and welfare, and/or financial), if she became incapacitated. But her husband was not happy with this. She was a high wage earner and had a separate bank account which the family wanted to access in order to pay bills, hence the safeguarding concerns.

In compiling the report, the IMCA used large drawings to understand the views and preferences of Petra in order to further a decision about whether she could return home or, alternatively, which nursing service she should use. Drawings showed where they were, and the IMCA spoke to her husband and Betty about this before researching and visiting services. Petra was able to express a preference for location. Regarding beliefs and values, Petra's husband was a Muslim and read the Koran to her in the hospital; in the view of her husband, Petra was also now a Muslim. This, for Betty, was unlikely as Petra had never shown any interest in religion previously. The IMCA reflected that it was possible that someone's views could change after a brain injury but was conscious that previous views should predominantly be taken into account. In one of the meetings of professionals—in fact, a best interests meeting requested by the IMCA—a spiritual assessment of Petra was considered as a way of determining what it was that sustained Petra in terms of well-being. The outcome was that an application to the Court of Protection to take control of Petra's finances was considered; however, the application did not need to go forward since the safeguarding situation was resolved with improved relations between parties (see further, Morgan 2011a).

1.1.2   Case Study 2: Alistair

Alistair was a 45-year-old Scotsman known to mental health services who was in a non-communicative state as a result of cardiac arrest resulting in a hypoxic brain injury. He was a music teacher who was popular with his students. He had loved working in the city, but recently colleagues thought his home was in disarray and that life had become confusing for him. On this occasion Alistair was admitted to a general hospital in a city and did not have cardio-pulmonary resuscitation (CPR) for at least 30 minutes. He was then taken to an Intensive Care Unit (ICU), where he underwent a tracheotomy and the introduction of a gastrostomy (feeding tube.) He was moved to a hospital for rehabilitation. The move from there was a best-interest decision but not straightforward as it depended on establishing what Alistair's wishes would be if he were able to state them and thus required an IMCA.

A dual-qualified Professional Advocate (mental health) and IMCA, was instructed in this case. As an IMCA, she chose to speak to Mrs Q., the mother of a student of Alistair's. Mrs Q. thought that Alistair's job and his niece in Canada were the most important things to him. Alistair's city-based colleague was asked whether he would wish to remain in this city and his job *or* go to live in Scotland close to a family friend. The balance of opinion from his far-flung family and friends was that he would wish to go back to Scotland. The IMCA had been involved in particular also because there were concerns following his cardiac arrest that some of his contacts had newly been exploiting him in the use of his home.

There were also issues about the transport from the city to Scotland and finding the appropriate service where Alistair could stay. This latter would have needed to be of a high standard in order to manage his tracheotomy and tube feeding process. Angus, a friend of Alistair's family, informed the IMCA that there was a local hospital near his home in a Scottish city which took people with complex needs. Since Alistair was no longer able to manage his own money, the IMCA recommended that consideration should be given regarding appointeeship for Alistair, to be arranged either through the local authority or in respect of an individual deemed appropriate to support and represent him in that. There had been no evidence of financial abuse. Alistair remained in the city area as he had some good contacts there.

The outcome was that Alistair remained in the city for the time being because there were concerns about his safety if he were to be moved a long distance with the tracheotomy and gastrostomy. The question about whether he could eventually move would be visited later. The IMCA suggested that a further care review referral should be made, and a mental health advocate colleague continued to support him with visits.

Before reflecting on these case studies, I wish to draw attention to IMCA training expectations which affect the way that these advocates reflect upon their practice.

1.2   Reflexivity and IMCA Training

Training for IMCAs requires employees to have the Independent Advocacy Qualification (IAQ) Level 3/4 Certificate and Diploma in Independent Advocacy; this began to quantify competencies which are needed to carry out the role illustrated in the above examples. For example, Action for Advocacy's competency matrix for Unit 305, which provided 12 credits for IMCA towards an overall qualification for Independent Advocacy via City and Guilds, included, for example, in 'Outcome 5: Work with People who Lack Capacity' the ability to 'use strategies to work with people with dementia...' (Action-for-Advocacy 2009). For this vocation-related qualification, obligatory for statutory advocates, candidates had to compile a portfolio of examples to demonstrate their skills. Reflective practice would be an important ingredient both in terms of training and qualifications and in relation to the case studies above. The 'reflexive process' is covered in educational literature, often influenced by Schön in his work, including *The Reflective Practitioner* (1983) (see also J. Brown and Libberton 2007; Davies 1999; McNiff 2002; P. Turner 2007 in relation to health and social care). Reflexivity is therefore a tool used to integrate material in a way which will satisfy not only the practitioner but also social care or advocacy theorists, spiritual care coordinators or practical theologians. This angle is certainly key, but in these cases I also want to show that reflexivity and reflection upon practice has impacted the outcomes which IMCAs and advocates experience in their work. Bolton offers this definition:

> Being *reflexive* is focusing close attention upon *one's own* actions, thoughts and feelings and their effects; (as distinct from) being *reflective* (which) is looking at the whole *scenario*: other people, the situation and place... (Bolton 2005, p. 7)

The IMCA has to be very reflexive in her/his role in establishing the wishes, preferences and best interests of a client. Sometimes this process will confirm the views of the decision-maker and at other times it will challenge them. Although not a social worker, the IMCA will share many skills with those in that professional role; however, as an independent interrogator of the process, which both medical consultants and social workers take forward, she/he occupies a unique place. Some IMCA training material clarified the specific interrogative role in report-writing, which the MCA ascribed to advocates:

> Auditing is an aspect of reports and focuses more on the process of the decision making, whether it is compliant with the Mental Capacity Act and should reflect how the decision meets the requirements of the best interest checklist and the principles of the Act. It therefore has a more legalistic aspect to it than the person centred style of report. (Action-for-Advocacy 2010, p. 18)

The Department of Health said it expects IMCAs to 'audit' the decisions about the move or treatment of someone unable to make decisions about these matters—for example, in supporting a client's move or in checking or challenging legally whether a particular medical procedure is meeting the client's needs. The cases above draw on the material used in the formal IMCA reports, which also show the auditing process underlying them. In short, then, the role of the independent advocate can be conflicted and 'common sense' may be a helpful category with which to describe the 'specialised person-centred approach,' independent of social work or medical professionals, which IMCAs are required to negotiate.

Cornwell spoke of challenging assumptions in the interaction between the medical and common-sense approaches in which the medical approach is usually, but not always, dominant (Cornwell 1984, p. 22). Advocacy practice over time is thus concentrated in what Schön has called the 'knack' or 'special feel for the ball' from the analogy of the baseball pitcher (Schön 1983, p. 54), which I want to link with the acquired skills of the IMCA. IMCAs reflect both in action and upon action, but especially as they negotiate space for clients or patients within a system which feels alien to the clients.

1.3   Reflections on the IMCA Case Studies

In the examples above, Petra and Alistair were individuals with different conditions resulting from an accident and cardiac arrest, respectively, and in different social situations, which may have had safeguarding implications. In these cases, the IMCA, who has from 2007 been available in safeguarding cases even if family exist, and advocate gathered information and fed it back to the decision-maker. Typically this involved a summary of what others said as well as insights from the IMCA's independent perceptions and reading of medical notes. The IMCA has a right to read these in order to consider a client's views and opinions. She/he also depends on information gained from contact with individual clients and from those close to them. In one case, the IMCA requested a best-interest meeting. The cases had significant cultural and social scenarios (e.g., the interest in golf, the connection with family, however difficult, or with a non-UK culture), which needed to be taken into account and which the IMCA was able to highlight. One of the examples happened to have 'spiritual dimensions': there was a question about whether Petra was being compelled to participate in religious discourse against her will. How did the involvement of friends and families from elsewhere feed into a decision for Alistair to remain in a certain area? Could the IMCA and advocate have done more? It can be seen from both cases how the IMCA informed her/himself by talking to friends and family about a decision, especially if the decision-maker did not think the family were representing the individual's best interests.

It could be argued that service-users with ABI are one of the most vulnerable of the various client groups which IMCAs work with. Those with dementia, mental health problems or learning disabilities often have some capacities or strategies which they use to communicate. ABI, at its worst, prevents people from communicating, and knowledge of the views and preferences of an individual with a brain injury are very difficult to discern. This is because minds and specifically brains change inalterably due to stroke and various other conditions. It would be challenging to decide, for example, whether Petra had genuinely changed religion. Who could make that judgement except Petra herself, and there was very little chance of finding that out from her? This is where knowledge of religious or spiritual assessment may be helpful, a resource which has been promoted by the Royal College of Psychiatrists (2010) and others, and one which does not need a spiritual practitioner to be carried out (Eagger 2005a; Royal-College-of-Psychiatrists'-Spirituality-and-Psychiatry-Special-Interest-Group-Executive-Committee 2010). For example, with the condition of Korsakoff's Syndrome (alcohol-related dementia), I found that there were very few specialist services in some boroughs which met the needs of these service-users in the UK—let alone how someone in the community may be supported once referral for formal hospital treatment ends, tending to define that individual as not suitable for further rehabilitation. This raised general questions about emotional and cultural security and support in the community, areas about which many, including generic advocates and often IMCAs, continue to be concerned.

2   The Growing Voice of the Advocate in Deprivation of Liberty Safeguards

2.1   London Borough of Hillingdon v Neary & Amor [2011] EWHC 1377 (COP) (9th June 2011)

I have referred above to the role of IMCAs in Deprivation of Liberty Safeguards (DoLS). The emergence of the IMCA role in public life has been underlined in a number of court cases, some of which have created important legal precedents. One of these was covered throughout the media, and raised the profile and enhanced the reputation of the service globally. The case, which was lost by the London Borough of Hillingdon, involved a dispute between Mark Neary and the council; he had asked for his autistic son, Steven, to go into respite care. Subsequently Steven was detained for a whole year in 2010 in his alleged best interests, and the detention was found to be unlawful under Article 8 of the European Convention on Human Rights—Right for Respect and Family Life. Originally, a referral was considered ineligible by the IMCA service, presumably because it was judged that Mr Neary could represent his son's best interests. When an IMCA was involved six months later, namely a section 39(d) IMCA, who was there to support the relative of a person deemed not to have capacity, it became a pivotal point in the case, along with the appointment of a solicitor who understood the legislation. This led to the judgement that the deprivation had been unlawful. The judge in the Court of Protection, which was unusually open to the public and press after pressure from the *The Independent* newspaper and because of the public interest, referred to the IMCA report as an 'impressive document' (EWHC 2011). IMCAs do not generally attend court but may do so; however, their reports may be used in court, as happened here. The IMCA, interviewed later for a radio programme, which weighed whether the DoLS process was too complicated and the referral take-up inconsistent across boroughs, and therefore in need of reform, explained her role:

> The first basic point was that Steven wanted to go home and it was not in the paperwork, and the first thing you look at when you do a Best Interests

decision is what does the individual want; because even if the individual does not have capacity, they may have views about your proposal, and that is really important. The Best Interests Assessor and the IMCA look to see whether it really is a deprivation of liberty. And one of the big things in a DoL is the family objecting to the restriction and it was not written in the paperwork. I thought the Court of Protection would slate them. If the Court of Protection got hold of the paperwork, the local authority could be in all sorts of trouble and that's what turned out to happen. (H. Barnes 2011)

The IMCA in this example had a straightforward part to play in supporting the case on its way to court. If the local authority decision-makers had had sufficient training it might not have happened. The judge applauded the attitude of Mr Neary in remaining level-headed, as well as the IMCA's work. It is evident from this example how the advocate applied her professional training and her background in advocacy to perform a common-sense role, albeit in underlining the importance of paperwork which meets the needs of the most vulnerable. Both Mr Neary as the carer, importantly, and the IMCA showed patience and balance, which could be described as desirable in terms of virtue ethics. For the IMCA this was part of occupational behaviours; for the carer and user of the service, Steven, it was his life which was affected, and that makes the virtuous triumph more commendable.

The evidence from interviews with individuals about advocacy will suggest that a virtue ethics approach, which I expand on below (6.2), could be useful in assisting advocates to reflect upon their practice. In explaining the nuances of 'common sense,' which I will bring in as a category in explaining how advocates saw their role, Ruth noted the need for the practitioner to distinguish between what may be *'patronising and disabling for a client and what may be empowering'* (See below 4.2.3). Furthermore the advocate herself should be able to reflect upon this process and balance reactions in an Aristotelian way, in order to maintain an effective relationship with a client. In the next section I group a number of cases together by theme.

3   Theme-Based Case Studies

3.1   Theme A: Advocacy Confronts Barriers of Stigma

'Well, if it was me, there on that bed, would you send me (away)?'
(Norah)

Angela (See Appendix 2) had recounted how she had been drawn into advocacy first as a volunteer, and how it then turned into a career for her. A friend had become unwell, she reported, and in the process of supporting him, she said, she…

> *became aware of how difficult it was for individuals to get the care, treatment, information that they needed, and what struck me very much in my own experiences of supporting him was how different his experience was when he went to meetings by himself from when I went to meetings accompanying him. And his experience was when he went to meetings by himself he received very little information, he wasn't listened to, um, he didn't get the responses to questions he was asking, um… he was knocked around from pillar to post. But, interestingly, whenever I attended meetings with him I would get responses. He would ask questions and they would respond to me, health care professionals would respond to me, and if they didn't answer his questions, and I interjected to prompt them to answer the question that he actually wanted to ask, they would respond. And it seemed to me quite ridiculous really.… (Angela 2007, October 1)*

Angela's advocacy practice was ultimately influenced by the experience of supporting a friend of hers, in 'informal advocacy,' in his encounter with the mental health system. This revealed a problem of residual stigma amongst some professionals. This friend stayed in Angela's flat, and she found that it was difficult for him to access support on his own. What struck Angela was… *'how different his experience was when he went to meetings by himself… he didn't get the responses to questions she was asking…'* (Angela 2007, October 1). Angela's friend was an outpatient, and she said that she thought that the professionals were on their best behaviour when she was around with him. These factors Angela found *'ridiculous'* and '*outrageous*' (Angela 2007, October 1). Angela was a quietly purposive and precisely spoken participant for whom these emotions were genuine.

Angela developed this point further in that her familiarity with her friend meant that she understood that he was asking '*perfectly reasonable questions, (and) trying to be as helpful as possible.*' These perceptions, in conjunction with the fact that this was her first experience of mental health services, led Angela to a conclusion that her friend's experience, if generalised, had implications for the state of mental health care and the benefits agency in the UK. She found their engagement with those with mental illness '*appalling*':

> *If this is how you treat someone who is being very reasonable, who... would very much like to engage with any help that is given, how on earth do you treat people who aren't able to be this helpful?* (Angela 2007, October 1).

Her reflection on the inadequacy of one mental health service in particular sustained Angela and influenced her in her approach to advocacy practice. This example showed how particular patients may be inadvertently or deliberately stigmatised or sidelined in their treatment. However, it was only one example, and I do not have evidence from the particular professionals involved to provide another side of the story. But what other evidence is there for similar experiences which people may have in accessing mental healthcare? There was evidence from spiritual care coordinators:

> *S: it was really interesting the way she was being spoken to and she was literally just, you know it was almost as if she wasn't a human being and she'd just been spoken at, and when I spoke up for her, the whole atmosphere changed in the ward round. They began to praise her, they began, you know, to affirm her and they gave her some freedom and she got everything she needed. ... and she was looking at me, and a complete change, change-around.* (Sarah and Karim 2008, December 4).

Here Sarah was speaking of a woman with a debilitating mental disorder for whom '*the whole atmosphere changed in the ward round*' due to Sarah's intervention. Sarah felt that it had been as if '*she wasn't a human being*' but following her own advocacy there had been a new release of praise, affirmation and freedom for the individual from staff. Karim commented on the theme of whistle-blowing, although the discussion was not framed in that way:

> *When there are a whole lot of patients from different wards and the information is triangulated I feel that there is something wrong, which might or might not be paranoid, then I have due concerns… (I say) 'What do you think about it?' and just make sure it is reported… see what their view is…*
>
> *F: Do you get a response?*
>
> *K: It's fairly recent, I had a response which amazingly was very much in support of my view.…* (Sarah and Karim 2008, December 4).

When asked about his experience of advocating for patients, Bernard mentioned that a regular client of his had had problems getting a copy of a letter sent to a general practitioner (GP) for herself.

> *Bernard: Well, today for example, there was somebody whom I see for counselling regularly who has had real problems in getting a copy of the letter sent to the GP, a copy for herself, which is her right, and I suggested she get in touch with PALS, which she has now done, and they were going to get back to her, um, because she just felt that the psychiatrist was just diverting away from her question, you know, 'I want a copy of the letters'… a lot of prevarication, you know it's really quite important. It's often a safe and reliable way of challenging, you know, inappropriate behaviour, or people feel confused about the treatment they are getting.* (Bernard 2008, August 19).

Although Bernard did not himself take action, he suggested that she should use a complaints process and supported her in that as she felt that *'the psychiatrist was just diverting away from her question.'* Bernard noted that getting a copy of a letter was a powerful way to address the confusion that people feel about the treatment they are getting (Bernard 2008, August 19). This technique whereby a patient may engage with his or her treatment through a GP and take control is related to direct engagement with a GP. This was an area in which Bernard provided a further example:

A Hindu patient who felt he was getting short shrift from his consultant and CPN, there were some rearrangements where people were moved into different teams to match GPs' surgeries but that for some people who had difficulties that took a very long time, so I supported him during that time. (Bernard 2008).

Bernard was asked to make a complaint about the patient's treatment whose diagnosis was *'borderline.'* When he agreed to do this because he knew him better than others, and did so, *'there was quite a lot of anger,'* according to Bernard, and although it was considered by his manager that it was *'entirely appropriate'* for him to be fulfilling this role, the National Health Service (NHS) Trust, Bernard's employers considered it not so. Direct challenge was another method used by an advocate to combat stigma. In this short example the wife of a self-advocate with learning disabilities who, according to her husband, looked *'a little bit disabled,'* was defended by another client in the face of discriminatory behaviour from schoolchildren:

My wife here was at a bus-stop and a crowd of school kids were taking the micky out of her so Laura went in and told them off so I think that Laura was acting like an advocate then. (Micky et al. 2008, May 14).

In this case the participant identified this as good advocacy practice. From learning disability advocates (and Norah in particular) there was evidence of systematic historical discriminatory behaviour.

You see when people were put into these long stay hospitals they were told not to keep in contact with their friends and relatives. They were advised that it was kinder and better to forget them. So those parents who maintained contact were strong if you like and challenged the system.... (A Norah and Bella 2009, December 14).

This counsel in favour of social stigma has been widely reported and is symptomatic of institutional discrimination against which advocates were in the forefront in exposing, for example, in the evidence that they pioneered the Person Centred Planning approach in 1984 (Bella

2010). Advocates reported that churches were not always havens of safety and anti-discrimination. Again, according to Bella, one advocacy client reported the following exchange although its veracity was questioned by Norah.

> B: And I said, 'Well, why do you feel that, other people go to other things, and she said, "Well when I went to St Peter's they didn't want me there they only wanted normal people."'

Norah said she could not believe them saying that, and Bella stated that that was what was heard anyway. Norah questioned whether it was reported speech (A Norah and Bella 2009, December 14).

Bella was actually questioning the 'chapel model' whereby people with learning disabilities who are not welcome in churches prefer to have spirituality brought to them. This was because they were felt to make a noise in some churches and had been made unwelcome there. This could have encouraged them to consider a socially exclusive approach to worship (in a chapel) rather than being part of a mainstream worshipping heterogeneous community. In the dialogue which ensued, it became clear that one particular church was being discussed. This was illustrative of the social and spiritual damage which institutional behaviours can cause and how advocates challenged and counteracted these. But a more personal example of this was also given by Norah. One of her clients needed treatment at Accident and Emergency and at first the doctor did not want to accept him because the long stay hospital he then resided at was not covered by that general hospital. Norah protested, as she put it in her own words:

> And I just said, 'Well, if it was me, there on that bed, would you send me to [name of hospital],' and he said, 'No, oh all right, I'll do it.' (A Norah and Bella 2009, December 14).

It turned out, following the procedure, that the injury the surgeon was treating involved a ruptured artery and that the service-user could have bled to death. As Norah said, her client was very 'precious' to her family. This was potentially a 'crime,' Norah stated, an act of discrimination which could have resulted in death or physical disability. Staff at the long stay hospital told of a similar accident when a patient with learning disabilities lost the use of a hand because of an alleged carelessly stitched '*botched*' job at a hospital.

The actions represented in this section belonged to the activity associated with advocacy, but not all the protagonists were employed as advocates. Nevertheless, all the examples could comprise 'equalising' activities, but especially those of Angela and Norah. Norah's '*strong identification*' with the service-user had a moral and spiritual significance which I will develop further below. I have looked at how practice addresses barriers of stigma; now I will consider aspects of the barriers of culture in relation to advocacy.

3.2   Theme B: Advocacy Confronts Barriers of Culture

'Getting people's views across feels rewarding' (Fauzia)

Fauzia, an Urdu speaker, provided a clear example from community advocacy (Fauzia 2007, October 1) of a culture barrier. She stated that people who had language barriers had particular problems accessing the help they needed, which could distress them. Although Fauzia may not speak the language, as an advocate she was able to organise an interpreter. Rather than only being concerned that people's words were translated, Fauzia wished to get '*peoples' views across to GPs… (which) feels really rewarding*'; when it was a language she understood she was irritated that people used her as a translator, '*when I'm not, I'm an advocate*' (Fauzia 2007, October 1). As a member of the same community with similar values to some of her clients, this advocate's approach was an example of how cultural capital in relation to mental health awareness was also used to overcome barriers of stigma within culture.

Nebi mentioned the advantages of the advocate role over his previous one as it was '*not a passive job, like an interpreter in which you only relay what is being said*' and enabled the advocate to have more freedom and more of a say in treatment of clients (Nebi 2007). The relationship between advocacy and interpretation was discussed further. El Ansari et al. (2009) argued that there was room for the professionalisation of bilingual advocates, that is, first language speakers who used their linguistic knowledge in healthcare advocacy. An earlier study heralding the Patient Advice and Liaison Service (PALS) argued insistently that:

> Mainstream services, including advocacy, must reach a minimum standard of cultural competence. This standard should address the five themes of identity, faith, racism, language and gender. The standard should be agreed at national level and should be a precondition for any statutory funding to the voluntary or independent sector. (Rai-Atkins 2002, p. 45)

It was also noted that there may be discrimination against these advocates by employers since they come from Black, Asian, Minority, Ethnic (BAME) groups, according to the cited articles. As I have argued, it has been difficult for independent advocacy to make its case in health and social care, but the advocacy which El Ansari et al. (2009) promoted was dissimilar because the advocates described were employed by trusts. It may be described as a form of advocacy, but it is probably not 'independent advocacy.' Independent advocacy and IMCA practice in particular would insist that the roles of translator or interpreter and advocate are distinct and independent to avoid conflicts of interest. No doubt, having an advocate with linguistic skills is helpful and may be more efficient, as Fauzia and Nebi showed, but experience demonstrated that keeping the two roles separate was more effective. In addition, the professionalisation of independent advocacy was probably at a more advanced stage than specialist bilingual advocacy, but the former may later have an impact on the development of the latter (El Ansari et al. 2009; Nebi 2007, October 22).

Nevertheless, the chaplain Zablon mentioned the advantages of an advocate understanding the mother tongue and culture of the speaker. An advocate can, he said, *'with the permission of the person, put it clearer.'* Zablon expanded to talk about the importance of direct experience, for example, through a family member having had mental health issues, and of common humanity as more important than clinical knowledge in the role (Zablon 2008, September 19). It was evident from Angela's testimony above and elsewhere that transparency in meaning is vital in discussions about mental health welfare and diagnosis, a matter of life and death. This was particularly true in the poignant example which Jana brought to the table. She occupied a dual role as an advocate and patients' council facilitator having begun her career as an administrator and advanced from that in the organisation:

> *reaching out to people who don't know about the service, or who… don't want to think about it… so they fear… a colleague of mine, she is supposed to be working with Polish people… not that there are no people, you know Polish people, with mental health problems, it's just that they don't talk about it… it's… quite important to actually find a way to actually reach these people.*
> (Jana 2007, October 22)

This example represented a double stigmatisation due to culture and mental health, one in which advocates were in a position to influence outcomes and in which they were active in trying to build bridges. The existence of this double or triple or quadruple disadvantage (if an individual had a physical disability and was from a hard-to-reach group) could also be shown from the example of Norah who described her work with people with learning disabilities and mental health as working with those with a *'dual diagnosis'* (A Norah and Bella 2009, December 14).

In summary, for some of those with mental disorders in England stigma and cultural factors have presented considerable barriers to receiving mental health treatment and social care. In my experience and research I found that advocates provided a nuanced and effective service in some places in London, and I identified ways in which these obstacles can be overcome for the well-being and enrichment of society. A controversial area was that of bilingual advocates, which, although such a service seemed to run counter to advocacy principles, could also represent an efficient means to meet cultural and linguistic support or treatment needs.

Another means to this end of combating disadvantage, I argue, could be a more focused attention to be given to cultural and spiritual needs and training, which I will deal with below. But firstly I will consider some of the ways that advocates and chaplains encountered barriers specifically in the mental health system.

3.3   Theme C: Advocacy Contests Psychiatric Opinion

'Important… to dig our heels in' (Revd Bernard A.)

I have previously mentioned the different kinds of advocates which exist within the sector. An IMCA would have to see someone based on a decision that a client lacked capacity in an area to consider what a best interest decision might be, and would necessarily be selective and focused when communicating with a client who lacked capacity. In many ways, an IMCA would be in a potentially more disempowered position than a standard mental health advocate, for mental health advocates are often under pressure to provide guidance or to support clients in resisting aspects of engagement with the psychiatric system. In order to locate these advocates correctly, I will rehearse the position which independent advocacy occupies within health and social care.

As touched on in the Introduction (1.5), there was evidence that social workers and other practitioners were in a good position to 'advocate' for their clients (Mallik 1998); however, advocacy was seen as a 'risky role to adopt' for nurses and not one which their career should embrace (Mallik 1997, pp. 130–135). If the 'central tenet of independence is missing from an advocacy relationship in which the advocate is also acting as a professional …' (Forbat and Atkinson 2005, p. 331) and if for a social worker it could also be problematic or bring them into conflict with their employers (Faust 2008, pp. 295–6; Gilbert 2010), the place of the independent advocate, in particular a mental health advocate, is to be active in this relationship. Atkinson stated that the rejection of the professionalisation of the role of nurse-advocate by the nursing elite left a gap to be filled (Atkinson 1999). This was the gap which voluntary sector organisations, funded increasingly by central government, were to fill. Thus independent advocacy came to be separated from 'the system' in order to better support and represent clients, patients or service-users, and this was particularly true in mental health.

The mental health advocates Angela and Nebi provided examples of how it was necessary to be a 'critical friend' in certain aspects of service provision as clients experienced it. I have provided some detail of Angela's personal challenge to the system on her friend's behalf (in

3.1, above). Angela also described the role of advocates as the process of encouraging mental health service-users to speak up and of providing clear information for them so that they can make decisions for themselves. She also subtly suggested that the advocates' role is to help service-users *'to think through what they are trying to achieve in relation to their mental health needs'* (Angela 2007, October 1). When asked about how an advocate would approach someone who was psychotic, Angela said that it was not her job to judge how much insight a person has, to make decisions on behalf of someone, or to be selective in the information that she presents to a client. In this sense there is a sharp difference between the role of the mental health advocate and the IMCA, which is emblematic of the difference between instructed and non-instructed advocacy. The two self-regulating questions Angela cited were:

> *a. Have I supported this person in the way they wish to be supported?*
> *b. Have I provided them with all the possible information to enable them to come to a decision at this particular moment in time?* (Angela 2007, October 1)

The two foremost desirable qualities for advocates which Angela mentioned (above) were the ability to listen and the ability to allow individuals to make decisions for themselves. At first Angela said that many people struggle with the first question, then she added that both questions were difficult. In relation to this desirability of autonomy, Nebi provided further evidence of how advocates would contest decisions made in wards. He spoke of his understanding of advocacy as an *'extension of the civil rights movement'* and the need to harness the energy of people who had been the *'victim of institutions'* within the occupation. In distinguishing the advocate's role from that of an information and advice worker, Nebi saw the mental health's advocate function as *'someone who takes what the service user says at face value and supports them... whatever fantasies they may have...'* He elaborated further:

> *you are already in a very good position not to give advice—not to act in the best interests approach—so at the end of the day you are doing different work... if someone is asking for discharge, you support them not because you know they*

are... well enough to be turned out but because they want it and you leave the judgement of whether they are well enough to professional doctors.... (Nebi 2007, October 22)

Nebi described the non-judgemental and affirmative line which advocates take in going with the flow of the client's wishes. He drew a distinction with medical 'best interests' which curtail freedoms and showed that advocates are in a position to assert the in-patient client's wish to be discharged. Nebi went into further detail about this negotiation process regarding discussions with a doctor about medication regimes and how, if a client felt a dose was too high, the advocate could pass that on and thus empower the client and make him a *force to be reckoned with.'* I asked if that was not something that could be done via the nursing staff on the ward.

N: Yes, it's completely impossible, I would say, with some of them with whom there is a good relationship... unless something goes wrong... they cannot have the same sort of relationship. (Nebi 2007, October 22)

Nebi illustrated that the point at issue was the discharge (whether it is voluntary or from a compulsory 'section') as an area of activity which advocates necessarily engaged with clients in the psychiatric system. Since detention, or deprivation of liberty, is technically a violation of a human right, clients needed support to question dosages and to attend mental health tribunals, one of the roles of IMHAs which grew out of generic mental health advocacy. Nebi felt that the challenge (*'it's completely impossible'*) to the system absolutely needed the support of an independent agent due to the fragility of relationships with staff in the institution, a point which Angela's experience echoed.

Asked about the contribution advocates made, Angela also reflected on the advocate's engagement with the mental health system:

... from straightforward issues by providing information at a particular time, to complex issues where people are being detained in situations which are potentially illegal... you are not necessarily able to change the treatment on behalf of the service user, but to challenge it... in challenging it they are able to come to

terms with it and understand it better. Often advocacy cannot get what the service user actually wants but they can ask questions...

Facilitator: ... Do you think the constant visiting can change the environment, the staff attitudes?

A: Again, it can do, but I think that's a bit of a mixed bag. It depends how good the advocacy service is. If it's a good advocacy service it can motivate staff to lift the bar and be more pro-active in providing good care and treatment and adhere to good practice and to ensure that patients are treated appropriately. But where an advocacy service is not functioning as well as it should do, doesn't have the respect of the staff, it can actually have the opposite effect. (Angela 2007, October 1)

Angela noted how advocacy can effect change for clients (who may be detained unlawfully) through challenging treatment and enabling clients to understand and come to terms with it, and recent legal case law (often based on the Human Rights Act) has shown how areas in which advocates work (e.g., DoLS following the Bournewood case) have undergone change. When asked about how the action of advocates can change the psychiatric environment, Angela argued here that an advocacy service can either raise the status of the occupation or bring it into disrepute. Ruth, another mental health advocate, also shared her views about the system:

... a lot of the time I'm thinking, 'Thank God I am not in your situation. I better keep myself safe. I mustn't get myself into this hospital, the services are really bad.' I think what goes on is many things but one of them is alarm actually. I think you can feel alarmed that someone in this society in this day and age has this experience so there is a tendency to want to make it better for this person cos in a way you want to make it better for yourself. (Ruth 2007, November 21)

Ruth showed personal concern about the state of affairs in some hospitals based on her previous involvement with clients, and drew attention to a motivation which may depend on a psychological need for a worker to be validated.

The ambivalence of particular services within psychiatry can be set alongside Angela's challenge to the system; this could be contrasted with criticism of advocacy itself from within the psychiatric literature, perhaps as a result of the poor practice which Angela mentioned above. For example, here Gamble (1999) accused advocates of condoning violence, an accusation which was then firmly rebutted (particularly in relation to accusations of violence) in the correspondence column of the 'Psychiatric Bulletin':

> I am concerned that the ethics of some advocacy movements are not those of doctors but that they may be using their access to vulnerable people (psychiatric patients), to promote their own anti-medical agenda... Local advocates have told ward patients that nurses are unable to fight back if attacked, a tacit encouragement of violence against staff.... (Gamble 1999, pp. 569b–570)
>
> Dr. Gamble expresses concern about the "anti-medical establishment political agenda" and "destructive ideology-driven power" of "some advocacy movements" — including, apparently, our own service. Dr. Gamble's use of terms such as political and ideology-driven we can forgive (and would be interested to debate further, in the context of mental health advocacy and the psychiatric system), but we take strong exception to the other labels he puts upon us. Our advocacy service operates in accordance with a policy drafted painstakingly over a period of some months.... (R. Smith et al. 2000, pp. 30b–31)

Advocacy practice, which was seen as beneficial by clients, was also perceived as a threat by some care workers and treated as suspect by some doctors, and was therefore a contested site. It should be noted that the defence of advocacy was based on what opponents would see as a very recently drafted and possibly suspect policy: on the other hand the fact that advocacy has been enshrined in law since that exchange in 2000 indicates that the actions of advocates had more weight and therefore would be more reflectively undertaken. Spiritual care coordinators do not align themselves with professional advocacy but see that they use similar skills.

Bernard recounted (see (c)) that patients were moved into different teams to match their GP surgeries, which caused one Hindu patient to want to make a complaint. As he said, *'it's quite important for us to dig our heels in and follow the complaint through really'* (Bernard 2008, August 19).

As far as general contact with staff was concerned, chaplains Bernard and Dorothy spoke about their involvement on psychiatric ward rounds as a comparatively rare occurrence. Dorothy said that she would not be looking *for that level of involvement*' unless there was a special situation and the patient gave permission for her to be there (Dorothy 2008, September 18). Bernard said that he would attend if a patient asked him to do so (Bernard 2008, August 19). Ethically this would also be true for a mental health advocate and for IMHAs although IMCAs would not need consent due to the permission being obtained through the best interests principles of the Mental Capacity Act.

Sometimes an advocate appeared to be of great benefit to the functioning of the mental health system. The chaplain Karim told the story of a patient who was very ill and whom he knew well:

> *the advocate knew this person as well... (and he) elected to keep contact with the advocate and severed all relationships with everyone who had ever worked on the ward and he had known previously....* (Sarah and Karim 2008, December 4)

As Karim put it, the advocate was the link-man and was entrusted with messages which he passed on to Karim. In this situation the advocate was exercising an empowering role in that he was espousing the cause of the client who instructed him independently of the NHS, including the chaplaincy, which the client may have perceived as compromised.

In this section I have considered advocacy practice and its capacity to challenge decisions in healthcare, especially in psychiatry. Advocacy seemed to be perceived as a contested site and was sometimes seen as 'anti-psychiatry'; on the other hand, there was evidence that the empowering and equality-based approaches of advocates pointed to models of practice requiring description, which I will consider further. For example, the position which Angela adopted in supporting her friend and the actions which the advocate (the 'link-man') took were ultimately supportive of the well-being of individuals for whom they were advocating.

4   The Extent and Limits

In this chapter I have described case studies from different advocacy practices including the particular role of the specialist IMCA form of advocacy in relation to people with ABI. I related this role, via the stories of the individuals, to indicators about specific IMCA training and reflective practice needs. I did so with the intention of broadening approaches to the best-interest enquiry process and showing how the awareness of advocates can embrace spirituality. In the DoLS-IMCA Court of Protection case, the wide range of possibilities within the MCA was set out, for example, with the deployment of a Sect. 39(d) IMCA. I consider that this reveals independent advocacy at its performative best, as well as the power of Steven Neary's father (his carer and principal advocate), as it laid down and asserted legislation for the improvement of the lot of the vulnerable and their relatives in what can be perceived as a hostile health and social care system.

IMCA guidance has stated that 'it is not possible for IMCAs to be able to know everything about a person when it comes to their beliefs or values.' It noted the importance of attempting to find out how their values (which is also true for wishes and preferences) can impact a decision. For example, 'if a person was born into a particular faith, do they still practise this?' If not, is this a choice or is it determined by circumstances—if, for example, they have been unable to leave the house for some time and have therefore been unable to attend a place of worship? Alternatively, according to the guidance, if they have or had non-religious, cultural or lifestyle-related beliefs and attitudes which have been integral to their identity, it would be important to investigate these in order to determine their relevance to the decision and ways in which they may be promoted or upheld for the client (Action-for-Advocacy 2011, pp. 34–5). In light of the above, it may be helpful for all healthcare professionals, IMCAs (and anyone working with or caring for those with ABI) to learn from the tools of spiritual assessment in relation to the most vulnerable clients, tools which are being used increasingly by spiritual care coordinators and some other staff in NHS hospitals and mental health trusts (see Eagger 2005a).

Through the theme-based case studies, I drew out how the practice was effective by describing how advocates approached power and took control with rights issues. Advocating dispositions accumulate, which are captured later in the terms Reconstructed Empowerment and Action Based on Equality. These are analytical descriptors for the skills I observed in advocates as they engaged with vulnerable individuals. In accordance with the argument, in this chapter I concentrated mainly on the second key question (Q2, Appendix 1) using a conceptual framework from all 'advocates' to explain the practice. Voiced testimonies above evidenced the consciousness of equality between human beings and the need to take a new perspective on uses of power in health and social care, which, I argue, is at the base of advocacy activity. Human equality is also foundational to spirituality, to Abrahamic faiths and to Practical Theology in the Christian tradition. A cluster of qualities and dispositions (formerly CRB-, *now* DBS-compliance [Disclosure and Barring Service], safeguarding ability and 'love for neighbour,' etc.) grow out of the engagement with advocates, their clients and chaplains, and further analysis of these in chapter (4.3.2) will follow. These constitute responses to Q1 with reference to aspects of Q3. I have also touched on responses to SQs to a large extent within the scope of the unfolding argument.

The current advanced state of independent advocacy has a significant back story. In the next chapter I consider the history and background from which the current practice evolved, returning in Chaps. 4 and 5 to a more analytical and reflective mode.

3

A History of Advocacy

1 Early Modern Times

1.1 Origins of Independent Advocacy

While a few have written on the history of self-advocacy and many more on mental health history, attempts to construct a history of independent advocacy as such are sparse (Bellamy et al. 2007; Bertram 2002; Rush 2004; Traustadóttir 2006). An ancient history of what could be described as 'advocacy' as a civil right in society may be discovered in an early 'ombudsman' role. From the Old Norse root, *umbodhsmadhr* meant a 'trusty manager' or 'commissary,' so that the ombudsman we know now commonly 'investigates complaints and mediates fair settlements, especially between aggrieved parties.' As a government official, especially in Scandinavian countries, s/he investigates citizens' complaints against the government or its functionaries (The-American-Heritage-dictionary 2000). In the UK NHS hospitals, PALS performs a similar role, and, since the 'A' in PALS originally stood for Advocacy, it may often be people who are less able to advocate for themselves for which such services are intended.

© The Author(s) 2017
G. Morgan, *Independent Advocacy and Spiritual Care*,
DOI 10.1057/978-1-137-53125-4_3

In the Ming Dynasty in fourteenth-century China, according to Ravich and Schmolka (1996), an ombudsman was mentioned as 'an appointee of the emperor to protect the people against his advisors and tax collectors,' who were usually his relatives. Professional (non-statutory) advocates support people with learning disabilities or mental health problems to make complaints. Although, strictly speaking, independent advocates are not involved in investigations of complaints, the Care Act 2014 widened the role in this respect, and the 2007 statutory expectations made independent involvement of IMCAs in the safeguarding process possible; this also may be the case when families and friends are ruled out of being able to support certain vulnerable individuals at certain times. The ancient Chinese 'protective measure' is not directly comparable to the safeguarding adults procedures, with which IMCAs are empowered to be involved, but it shows the continuity of a similar social role from an ancient and different culture (Fairbank et al. 1998, pp. 72–73; Gorczynska and Thompson 2007; Ravich and Schmolka 1996). Turning to Eastern monotheistic faith-based examples and mainstream religious teaching, for example, Christ's Sermon on the Mount (Matthew: 5–7, Bible), the Parable of the Final Judgement (Matthew 25:34–40, Bible) or the commandment to give alms (Sura 2:40, Koran) from the Christian and Muslim traditions, respectively, enjoined care for the most vulnerable. These comparisons show how the role of advocates is also deeply pastoral in welcoming disabled and vulnerable people. Drawing on the philosopher Macintyre (1999), Bretherton summarised the importance of the humanitarian motivation in social care:

> The practice of hospitality and what is in effect love of neighbour is learnt by due care of the disabled and dependent in one's community. It is through encounters with them that we discover errors in practical reason… and in the norms in our community… thus the community is better able to transform its reasoning and practices so as to enable all its members to flourish and all its relations… to be characterised by just generosity. (Bretherton 2006, p. 98)

Based on Aristotelian ethics, human flourishing and well-being can be linked with faith-based communitarian ideals and these are important themes in this explanatory study of the role of advocacy. In the next sections I consider spiritual and theological factors in the development of mental health advocacy.

1.2   Emergent Civil Rights for 'Lunatics' in Seventeenth-Century England

Some historians have located the origin of independent advocacy in the UK in the seventeenth century—a period in which civil rights were emerging—in a number of accounts of mental health development and advocacy. Nearly all of these derived from Brandon (1991), who was frequently cited, although it has not been possible to find a primary source for the following, either from further research or parliamentary records (Roberts 2008). In 1620 the House of Lords was thought to have received the 'Petition of the Poor Distracted People (or Folk) in the House of Bedlam.' This was a corporate complaint raised by inmates of the Bethlem Asylum against their inhumane treatment. They were forced to 'entertain' the public in exchange for food and clothing and were frequently shackled and subjected to other forms of physical 'treatment' and restraint (Brandon and Brandon 2000, p. 6; MIND 2008). I examine this pre-Enlightenment example of what would now be called 'human rights abuses' further, to support the link between the petition and the early advocacy tendency as well as to discern the cultural thread in the narrative. I will briefly consider the history of this institution, from its earliest days, a unique example in England.

Founded in 1247 and confiscated by Edward III in 1375, the original priory of St. Mary of Bethlem was used for 'lunatics' from 1377, but further details regarding the history of asylums are available elsewhere (Jones 1972). After the Fire of London, Robert Hooke was appointed city surveyor and designed the new (Bethlehem Hospital) in Moorfields, which opened in 1676; before this it only had around 30 patients, but by 1704 had 130. (It was replaced by the St. George's Fields Bethlem in 1815, now the Imperial War Museum; and in 1930 the new Bethlem Royal moved to its present site in Bromley, Kent.) From this limited evidence, the 'distracted folk' who could have presented the petition of 1620 would not have been numerous but could have been well-supported (even effective) 'self-advocates'; the fact that their identities are unknown indicates that they were probably neither rich nor well known.

At the door of the Moorfields Bedlam, the visitor was confronted, according to Roberts (1981a), with sculptures commissioned from the Danish sculptor Caius Gabriel Cibber (1630–1700), one of melancholia, the other of raving madness. These 'brazen, brainless brothers'[1] are now sited in an exhibition space inside the entrance to the Bethlem Royal Hospital, Bromley, see Fig. 3.1.

Roberts wrote that 'those who pass a theatre or a strip-joint today are tempted in by photographs of the performance. This drama had a

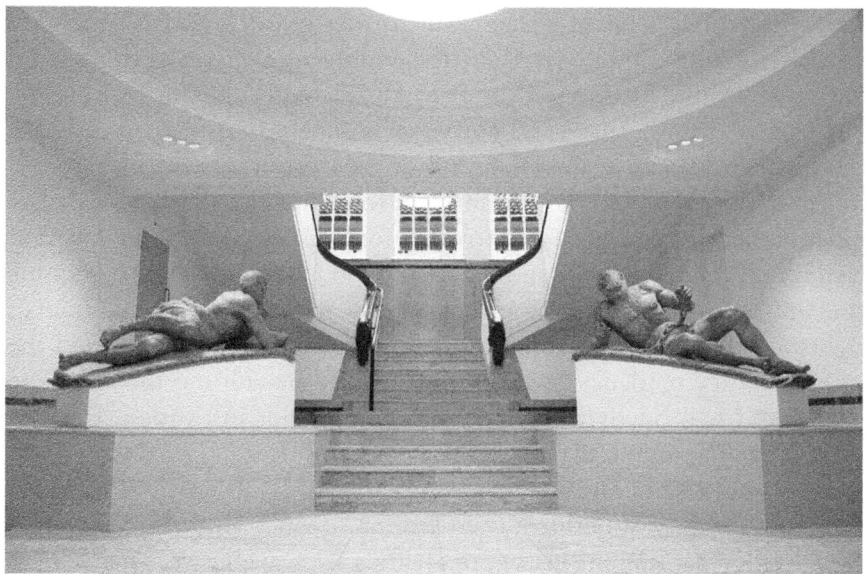

Fig. 3.1 'Melancholia and Raving Madness' by Cibber

---

[1]Close to those walls where Folly holds her throne,
And laughs to think Monroe would take her down,
Where o'er the gates, by his famed by father's hand
Great Cibber's brazen, brainless brothers stand;
One cell there is, concealed from vulgar eye,
The cave of poverty and poetry.
The Dunciad Book the First, Alexander Pope.

hundred year run and its actors were involuntary exhibits.' Until 1770 'lunatics' here were displayed to holidaying Londoners, for a fee, along with zoo animals at the Tower of London. Revulsion at such spectacles, due to a pricking of moral and spiritual conscience, and the burgeoning of a civil rights agenda in the seventeenth century, was already being noted (Roberts 1981a/1377 & 1666 & 1930).

Tryon (1689) spectacularly pinpointed the lack of a civilised and compassionate spirit at that time:

> It is a very indecent, inhuman thing to make... a show... by exposing them, and naked too perhaps of either sexes, to the idle curiosity of every vain boy, petulant wench, or drunken companion, going along from one apartment to the other, and crying out; this woman is in for love, that man for jealousy. He has over-studied himself, and the like...the poor creature falls a raving... and so the holy and tremendous name of God is dishonoured, whilst the wicked people, who think it is a diversion, instead of trembling as indeed they ought, being themselves really guilty of all these blasphemies... fall a laughing and a hooting... (Tryon cited in Roberts 1981d/1666)

The acutely observed guilt of the author as a voyeur of suffering, together with his sense that such spectatorship represented a breach of public and spiritual order (under the awe-inspiring watchful divine eye), was an early example of what would much later become stock-in-trade: in eighteenth- and nineteenth-century changes in the law and in rights-based and patient-centred approaches to health in the late twentieth century. The visceral desire to address the want of dignity and respect for a fellow human being, taken as an offence (blasphemy) against the divine, was later apparent in the campaigning agenda for equality and justice inherent in independent advocacy (Hervey 1986).

The single mention of the Petition is also often included as a significant early development in terms of the history of the 'survivor' or 'user movement' within mental health, which has parallels with the development of independent advocacy, especially mental health advocacy and self-advocacy (Brandon 2007; Brandon and Brandon 2000, p. 6). The 'holy discomfort' felt by Tryon in his seventeenth-century observations in England was followed by more active interventions, closely related to the definition we have drawn up as constituting advocacy. A comparison with what was happening elsewhere in Europe will help to slot these humanitarian and spiritual concerns into the Practical Theology category in which my book falls.

1.3   Emergent Civil and Political Rights for 'Lunatics' in Seventeenth- and Eighteenth-Century France

In a history of mental health nursing, Walk (1961) indicated 'the glorious work of St. Vincent de Paul and Ste. Louise de Marillac at St. Lazare in seventeenth-century Paris' with what we would now call those with personality (as well as mental) disorders (Walk 1961). French practices were considered to be advanced compared with treatments in England at that time (Rush 2004, p. 315). From a Roman Catholic theological perspective, de Paul taught his helpers that their work was more meritorious when they derived least satisfaction from it and when they were doing good in secret to patients who showed no gratitude. This happens to embody a clear instruction for Christian practitioners (Matthew 6:4, Bible). When Ste. Louise de Marillac, directress of de Paul's order of the Daughters of Charity, took charge of the nursing of the 'insane and senile patients at the Petites Maisons,' de Paul admonished them:

> Say to your selves 'I am going to honour in my patients the incarnate wisdom of God, who willed that He himself should embrace this state in order to sanctify it like all others.' (Walk 1961, p. 2)

From a philosophical perspective, in his cultural history, Foucault (1967) was both positive and critical about de Paul's view of the sacred state of madness. This 'lowest point to which God submitted in His incarnation,' in Foucault's terms, grew from the relatively healthy conception and space given to madness in the Renaissance and its 'instructive value.' However, in the following century the Church—and de Paul in particular—found in human madness the guilty innocence of the 'animal.' Foucault meditated on the liberty of madness against the background of Unreason or *déraison* (Fr.) and described 'classical rationalism' as guarding against unreason. Confinement, the 'birth of the asylum' and the eighteenth-

century medicalisation of mental health, including the work of the morally motivated, were viewed ambivalently by him (Foucault 1967).

Jean-Baptiste Pussin (1746–1811) worked for the classical 'alienist'
Philippe Pinel as the Chief Nurse or Superintendent of the Bicêtre asylum in France. Alienists were a group who held positivist views on madness and its physicalist cause (Hervey 1986, p. 248). Rush (2004, p. 315)
showed how Pussin had suffered from depression himself and recruited
staff from convalescing patients in the belief that, because of their experiences, they were able to provide the humanity and kindness needed
in a 'moral management approach' (as cited in Walk 1961, p. 3). Pinel
described these recruits as

> averse from cruelty through the recollection of what they had themselves
> experienced, and disposed to humanity and kindness from the value which
> for the same reason they could not fail to attach to them. (Walk 1961, p. 3)

Pinel's words and actions are a very clear example of an early form of
spiritually-motivated peer advocacy. Later Pussin was seen as pioneering
in relation to reform efforts, setting aside the use of chains as restraints
for his patients in 1798 and 1801, although these were replaced by 'strait-
waistcoats' (Walk 1961; Rush 2004).

While these insights were drawn from the early social history of mental
health nursing, and could be related to the role of nurse as advocate, they
also apply to the attitude demanded now in the role of an independent
advocate. Principles of vocation, empathy and what is contemporarily a
'patient-centred approach' were foremost in de Paul's account. For this
reason, amongst others, they can broadly be seen as religious as well as
empowering and egalitarian principles. I will examine the patient-centred
approach further in the accounts of twentieth-century advocacy.

Following the revolution in France (1789), in March 1790 a French
mental health revolution took place. A decree went out that within six
weeks 'all persons detained in fortresses, religious houses, houses of correc-
tion, police houses, or other prisons, whatsoever… so long as they are not
convicted, or under arrest, or not charged with major crimes, or confined
by reason of madness, will be set at liberty.' The 'mad' were to be examined
and either set at liberty or 'cared for in hospitals indicated for that purpose.'

In Paris arrangements were made for insane men to be sent to the famous Bicêtre and insane women to the Salpétrière institutions. (Two hundred insane women moved there in 1792.) After an initial period of confusion, the two institutions became reserved for the insane (Roberts 1981a/1789).

1.4   Emergent Political Rights for 'Lunatics' in Eighteenth- and Nineteenth-Century England

A further example of the French 'moral management approach' was pioneered in England by William Tuke. Moral management related to the French meaning of *la morale* as related to morale or emotional well-being rather than morality in terms of rights and wrongs. As a Quaker, Tuke advocated retreats and that the mentally disordered should be treated as members of a family with accordant responsibilities and privileges. This has been regarded by Sumner as one approach which had generally few if any defects in the history of psychiatry. The Retreat still exists today as a private mental health service in York, which is commissioned and used by other services (Sumner 1993; Tuke 1813). Tuke and others were involved in a campaign to improve conditions in the York Lunatic Asylum as opposed to his own private 'madhouse.' The visiting of female patients at the York asylum began in 1814 following reforms carried out by Tuke. This had involved the dismissal of all staff and the institution of a visiting programme by 'ladies,' and one in particular who had argued that female wards should be 'inspected by well educated persons of their own sex'; eventually members of Tuke's family carried out visits (Sumner 1993).

There is also evidence that a number of other leaders in English asylums protested against treatment and conditions within them. One 'alleged lunatic,' James Tilly Mathew, was active in 'self-advocacy,' asserting himself to be sane, in order to seek discharge from Bethlem. Although he was unsuccessful, the 'alienist' responsible was dismissed without a pension in 1816 (cited in Brandon and Brandon 2000, p. 6; Haslam and Porter 1988; Monro 1758).

It was not until later in the eighteenth and nineteenth centuries in England, following trains of events leading to the passage of the Lunacy Acts (1845 and 1890), that activities took place which can be identified both as political and social rights claims, and the heritage of present-day independent advocacy. Roberts (1981a) records that the 1890 Act was a major consolidating Act which remained the core of English and Welsh legislation until it was repealed by the 1959 Mental Health Act. The major change (in 1889) was that private patients, apart from chancery lunatics whose cases were dealt with by the Court of Chancery, should not be detained without a judicial order or 'reception order' from a Justice of the Peace. Roberts (1981a) wrote that 'pauper patients already required an order from the magistrates to be detained – although that provision was probably originally an authorisation of public funds rather than a safeguard of liberties as the reception order was intended to be' (Roberts 1981a/timeline 1890).

The 'reception order,' which was an early form of mental health section or DoLS, lasted one year. A medical report had to be sent to the Lunacy Commission before its expiry to request extension 'for another two years, then another three years, then another four years, then five years and thereafter at five year intervals' (Roberts 1981b/Section 38). Additionally, a thirteenth-century statute: *De Praerogativa Regis*, trans. 'On the King's Prerogative,' gave the Crown custody of 'the lands of natural fools and wardship of the property of the insane during their insanity.' This was the basis for their later management by the Lord Chancellor in the eighteenth century, for the title of 'Chancery Lunatics,' the existence of a judge called a 'Master in Lunacy' (from 1845) and 'Chancery Visitors' (from 1835). The current Court of Protection, which with its antecedents is considered one of the oldest courts in England, and the Court of Protection visitors, and conceivably independent advocates, all had their origins here. A law of 1890 also distinguished between the responsibility for an individual's property and his/her person, a distinction which exists up to the present in powers of attorney and deputyship (formerly receivership) (Roberts 1981c/Glossary Chancery Lunatics).

Therefore, in the early nineteenth century France was advancing towards a political and even social enshrinement of rights as advocacy and spiritual values, whereas England at a similar stage was only progressing slowly with civil rights awareness in some strata of society. In comparison with France, there was a lesser tradition of nursing by recruits drawn from former patients in England, where the approach was more akin to 'moral treatment' and 'social control,' according to Rush (Rush 2004).

Nonetheless, one example, of user involvement, cited by Rush (2004), was found in the establishment of the Alleged Lunatics Friends Society (ALFS) by John Perceval in 1845 (M. Barnes and Bowl 2000).

1.5   Political and Social Rights and Advocacy in England: The Case of John Perceval and the Alleged Lunatics Friends Society (ALFS)

Perceval had himself been confined in a 'madhouse' but, on his recovery, wrote about his experiences and encouraged others to share their views within the society and to protest at the persistence of inhumane treatment in so many institutions. However, as Rush (2004) noted, citing Brandon (1991), a limiting factor was that Perceval and others writing about their experiences in the nineteenth century came from the aristocracy rather than the poorer classes. The voices of the majority of people inhabiting institutions for the insane remained silent, according to Rush (p. 315), evidencing how England was second to France in this respect.

On the other hand, as Hervey (1986) showed, after the autobiographical stage following his psychosis, Perceval was part of a pressure group or movement which, although aristocratic in make-up and with many weaknesses, had some success at the heart of British society in improving conditions for all. Hervey also showed the struggle by Perceval against the upper class stigmatisation of 'lunacy' and the economic preference of some for their mentally ill (pauper lunatic) family member to live in county asylums rather than lunacy wards in workhouses. The county asylum had been introduced by Shaftesbury: a whole family rather than an individual could be confined there, and indeed the same choice was exercised by pauper lunatics themselves. There was evidence that those with financial or family support were cared for, with new top-down energy to give voice to the silent and disenfranchised, who were not (Bartlett 1998; Hervey 1986). It will be pertinent to examine the case of Perceval in some more detail as a prelude to an understanding of advocacy in the light of an active contemporary user movement.

The arguably 'outstanding example of advocacy' which Perceval set meant that he was attested in the history of the practice as a founder of the movement (Brandon and Brandon 2000, p. 6). The son of the only British Prime

Minister to be assassinated, Spencer Perceval, John was nine years old when this took place. His struggle with mental ill health was recounted in his 'spiritual autobiography' following a move to Paris and a meeting with Dr. Esquirol (in the lineage of Pinel, above). Esquirol advised him about political actions needed to reform the lunacy laws (Brandon 2007, p. 37). The memoir was released in two parts, in 1838 and 1840, and was seen as a foundation document in the history of mental health advocacy. Revealingly entitled

A narrative of the treatment experienced by a gentleman, during a state of mental derangement; designed to explain the causes and nature of insanity, and to expose the injudicious conduct pursued towards many unfortunate sufferers under that calamity (Perceval and Bateson 1962)

the Prefaces to Perceval's volumes contained what may be called 'advocacy manifestos.' He wrote:

I open my mouth for the dumb... I entreat you to place yourself in the place of those whose suffering I describe... Feel for them; try to defend them. (Brandon 2007, p. 39)

In the second part, the self-described 'attorney-general of all Her Majesty's madmen' (Gault 2008, p. 463) became more engaged:

I resolved – I was necessitated – to put my strength and abilities against that system, to fail in no duty to myself and to my country... to expose and unravel the wickedness and the folly that maintained it, and to unmask the plausible villainy that carried on. (Brandon 2007, p. 39)

In Hervey's (1986) measured assessment, the ALFS' ends—namely, to reduce illegal incarceration of patients, to improve conditions in asylums, to remind the public of their Christian duty and to forward matters overlooked by the Lunacy Commission—were hampered by their limited means and their understandable alliances with radical politics and the Chartist movement. Since Chartists campaigned against property-based suffrage, potential supporters in the elite found ALFS less sympathetic. Due also to its maverick and avant-garde 'patient-centred' approach, the ALFS probably had no more than 60 members. However, it received regular help from liberal-minded parliamentarians (Hervey 1986, pp. 253–4) and took up the cases of at least 70 patients between 1845 and 1863 (Hervey 1986, p. 262). Generally the society did not constitute a social movement but contained within it, in the displays of campaigning individualism and by virtue of some political success, the seeds of practices which have grown to be part of the mental health advocacy and statutory advocacy movements today.

For example, in 1853, ALFS wanted patients' legal rights displayed in the wards of every asylum. They wanted it to be recorded if patients disagreed with their diagnosis; they were concerned to safeguard patients' property by placing a seal on it; and they wished for half-way houses for those being discharged. It succeeded only in improving medical certificates and with an order for a coroner's report to be given in the case of a suspicious death (Hervey 1986, p. 258). Accesses to information, legal representatives and for a second medical opinion were obtained from the Lord Chancellor on three occasions in 1854 (Hervey 1986, p. 264).

Hervey referred to the interest shown by the Law Amendment Society (who fed into the Report on the Committee on Equity on the Law Respecting Lunacy in 1848) as being attributable to Perceval. Demands made by ALFS, some of which were successful, included requirements for a 'judicial' person to visit every patient after admission, because they were often refused access to an attorney or their presence in an asylum was kept from their friends; enforced residence conditions on asylum proprietors, after Perceval suggested juries should adjudicate on admissions; and for greater attention to be given to single people (Hervey 1986, p. 265).

When an heiress was placed in an asylum to stop her from giving her inheritance to a religious sect, and the judge, Chief Baron Sir Frederick Pollock, ordered that no person should be confined on the grounds of mental illness unless they were a danger to themselves or others in 1849, ALFS were interested because they hoped it would end the incarceration of harmless chronic patients including 'epileptics and idiots.' Much work was concerned with those who were unable to get help for themselves. It is possible to see the Pollock judgement as a precursor of the MCA principle that someone cannot be deemed to lack capacity because they made or are making an unwise decision (Hervey 1986, p. 262; Chancellor 2007, p. 19).

Hervey noted that ALFS uniquely brought test cases to court, having researched more equitable systems in France, Belgium and Prussia, and in this area of civil liberties, which most Victorians in the UK denied needed addressing. Perceval wanted to see local clergy visiting asylums; they would not come in 'representing the locks and keys which separate the patients from society, but come in as part of the neighbourhood, and repeat a little of the gossip of the day, and it would seem to supply a connexion with society' (Hervey 1986, p. 267). ALFS saw regular admission of the clergy and public as a real safeguard against abuses, and, in relation to this study, such discussion indicated a bond between advocacy and spirituality on account of Perceval's persona. Early 'safeguarding' problems were bolstered by Mill's criticism in 1859 of the 'contemptible and frightful evidence' (cited in Hervey 1986, p. 275) on which people were declared unfit to manage their own affairs. When in 1866, Perceval's nephew became the Lord Chancellor's secretary and then secretary of the Lunacy Commission, Perceval gained some peace of mind. It can be seen that Perceval and the ALFS made progress in patients' rights, asylum care and medical accountability, all of which are also integral concerns to advocacy practice (Hervey 1986, p. 275).

This present study will examine some of the cultural and religious themes in relation to the current practice of advocacy which Perceval commended as part of his analysis of the defects of Victorian mental healthcare. Brandon (2007) successfully countered the position taken by some that advocacy had its beginnings more recently in the 1960s, which Gault (2008) and Hervey (1986) bear out. Closer analysis of John Perceval's work and example showed that the seeds of independent advocacy had been planted long before the civil rights and social reform movements, which were part of the development of advocacy in the second half of the twentieth century. It is to that era we must now turn and briefly to what led up to this.

2   Modern, International and Social Movements

With very little progress in the standard asylums in the second half of the nineteenth century in England, compared perhaps with that in specialist hospitals, the era of mental hospitals and institutionalisation gradually gave way to forerunners of community care, and created space for new examples of advocacy. The 1890 Lunacy Act was seen as consolidating previous acts—to which John Perceval and ALFS were precursors—until, after social rights legislation such as National Insurance (1911), Old Age Pensions (1918) and the Mental Treatment Act 1930, it was finally repealed in 1959, with a new Mental Health Act. This was a period described as one of 'therapeutic pessimism' in which the mentally disordered were contained, until the outpatient revolution of the 1950s. In 1930 there had been practically no outpatients, but their numbers grew as the demand for psychiatric beds fell, and by 1959 there was an increase to 144,000 attendances at outpatient clinics (Maclay cited in H. Freeman 1998; Roberts 1981a/1959).

2.1   Tides of Change

2.1.1   Self-Advocacy

I have considered Brandon's studies and contributions from a number of others to date the origin (above) of an advocacy 'tendency' much earlier than generally considered (Ravich and Schmolka 1996; Brandon and Brandon 2000; Brandon 2007). However, advocacy is generally perceived as a child of the civil rights' and social movement climate of the 1960s. A number of writers identified Scandinavia of the late 1960s as the opening of the modern era of (self-) advocacy. According to Traustadóttir, 'young people with learning difficulties met in social clubs to discuss their lives' (Traustadóttir 2006, p. 175). It was in Sweden that a group of people with learning disabilities drew up a list of requests about how their services should be provided, which was then passed on to decision-makers (Grant 2005, p. 159). Denmark saw the origin of 'systematic presentation of the normalisation principle,' namely that people with a learning disability should lead normal lives as opposed to living, for example, in residential accommodation (Gates 2002, p. 532). The Swedish National Conferences of Retarded Adults in 1968 and 1970 (Grant 2005, p. 160; Wolfensberger 1972, pp. 184, 189–193) were seminal, and in parallel the movement reached the USA in 1966 with a conference for parents of children with cerebral palsy in Pennsylvania. What had been recognised as a 'grassroots movement' began to find its full expression, including some international dimensions (Atkinson 1999, p. 5; Forbat and Atkinson 2005, p. 326; Brandon, Brandon and Brandon cited in Sim and Mackay 1997; Dybwad and Bersani cited in Traustadóttir 2006).

Marshall (1973) and Giddens' description of the continuum of progress from civil rights (eighteenth century), and then to political and social rights in the nineteenth and twentieth centuries, is helpful to analyse the process. Rights to economic and social security, education, housing and pensions brought with them the ideal of social citizenship, which advanced the notion of equality for all (Giddens and Birdsall 2001; Marshall 1973). This was a key principle in the ethos of disability rights and self-advocacy as well as in traditional Jewish and Christian religion and spirituality, for example, to love one's neighbour as oneself.

A history of the emergence of advocacy in the twentieth century therefore cannot ignore the rise of self-advocacy amidst the social ferment of the 1960s, with its emphases on civil, women's, gay and disability rights, and concomitant protest politics. The self-advocacy movement was significantly related to the larger disability movement, according to Traustadóttir (2006), and after marginalised and powerless groups began to reclaim their rights and freedoms (see also Evans 1979; J. Freeman 1975; M. Oliver 1990; Shakespeare 2006):

> Many of the first self-advocacy groups were established by former residents of large state institutions – often helped by staff, parents and other allies. They were often closely related to the fight to close institutions and demands for the right to live in the community. At the time people with learning difficulties were not seen as capable of articulating, or indeed understanding, their own needs and wishes. Others were seen as being better suited to speak and make decisions on their behalf. (Traustadóttir 2006, p. 175)

2.1.2   Social Rights and New Social Movements

The American and other civil rights and feminist movements of the 1960s and 1970s, the anti-nuclear and ecological movements of the 1980s, and other rights movements of the 1990s have also been characterised as 'new social movements' standing aside from the political process (Crossley 1999, 2007; Crossley and NetLibrary 2006). It is a 'paradox' of democracy, that voting processes are somewhat subverted, Giddens argued, so that more than ever before people were supporting social movements rather than using conventional political routes as a way of highlighting complex moral issues and putting them at the centre of social life (Giddens and Birdsall 2001, pp. 439–441). The emergence of user involvement—patients or citizens having an increasing say in their treatment or civic decisions—alongside 'the politics of participation' was facilitated by the state and the 'political opportunity structures' it created, as well as by social movements pressing for change. Moreover, the contemporary interest in user involvement was also associated with what has been identified as 'DIY social policy' (Klein and Millar 1995) according to Martin (2000). For him, Millar (1996) described how users mixed and matched services to meet their own care needs by the selection of specific providers, both from public and private sectors (Millar 1996, p. 191). This was later to lead to individual budgets, personalisation and what in 2008 emerged as 'self-directed support.'

The passion and involvement of users or former users of, for example, the mental health system has been referred to above and can be seen as an important socio-political trajectory, both in peer advocacy and its exemplification in eighteenth-century France by Pussin, as well as in emergent self-advocacy. It has commanded enthusiasm and a following of a quasi-religious nature. The notion of the patient as consumer or client, and 'consumer advocacy,' seen above (Ravich and Schmolka 1996) and in other literature (D. o. H. (DoH) 1995; Funk et al. 2006), built in the last 30 years. It culminated in the rise of the 'user movement' itself, which was strong in mental health but not confined to that sector (Pilgrim and Waldron 1998; Ridley and Jones 2001; Wistow and Barnes 1993). It is to that new social stream in mental health—the 'user' movement, members of which sometimes described themselves as 'survivors'—and its relationship to advocacy that I now turn.

2.1.3   User Movements and Professionalised Advocacy

In a chapter entitled 'Community Mental Health Promotion,' Tudor (1996) bracketed together the user and the advocacy 'movement' (Tudor 1996, p. 129). His review of the user movement in the 1980s and early

1990s covered how a receiver of mental health services has ranged in description from 'patient' to 'survivor.' The term survivor was picked up by 'Survivors Speak Out,' a user organisation founded at a Mind (the UK mental health charity) conference in 1985 representing 'survivors' of the mental health system. Favoured by Tudor, the term, 'user' was value-free and used in Italy (Italian *utenti* = users) where the mental health system was positively assessed by the author for its Democratic Psychiatry movement (Tudor 1996, p. 135), whereas 'consumer' carried the implication of choice, which was not always realistically there. However, with the introduction of 'individualised budgets' in some areas in England, this assertion needed to be revised. What had become a standard term, 'a person with mental health problems,' was critiqued for 'its libertarian value, disguising the very real differences between people' (Tudor 1996, p. 130).

Tudor then considered the two dimensions of advocacy. He cited Sang and O'Brien (1984), who, on the one hand, linked self-advocacy and citizen advocacy with the 'user trajectory' as a grass-roots phenomenon. Patient and independent (professional advocacy), on the other hand, were warned against as 'top-down' and inherently liable to lead to a 'take-over of the former forms of advocacy by professionals' (Sang and O'Brien 1984; Tudor 1996, p. 130). Wolfensberger, a founder of the advocacy movement, as Harrison and Davis (2009) noted, believed it was not enough to speak on behalf of another, but that advocacy 'implies a vigor [sic], a vehemence, a commitment... a high cost, often in the form of risk,' with concomitant 'hostility from others, taunts, being considered foolish or crazy, loss of income, loss of job, loss of health, physical hurt and violence – perhaps even (the risk of) death.' (Wolfensberger cited in T. Harrison and Davis 2009, p. 58). This energetic language was indicative of both a spiritual dimension to advocacy and systemic conflict by which such advocacy is characterised.

This clash of dimensions was one of many in the area of health and social care and advocacy illustrating the endemic creative tension. Articles on advocacy in nursing practice (as opposed to independent advocacy) constituted a sub-theme in the material (Vaartio et al. 2006; Watt 1997; Willard 1996). There were, of course, cross-overs and a danger that the term 'advocacy' had become either a portmanteau term meaning whatever the subject wanted it to mean—this was named by Wolfensberger (1977) as 'cheese advocacy' in the way that cheese can be added to any food (T. Harrison and Davis 2009, p. 58)—or, ultimately, that it lost value because it was redefined out of existence, for example, in the separation into 'dementia advocacy,' 'independent advocacy,' 'self-advocacy,' and so on. In addition to this, the validation deriving from the commissioning of IMCA (and, from April 2009, IMHA) service provision, brought with it a suspicion of collusion with the statutory sector on the part of other voluntary sector employees and pinpointed some disputed areas which need exploring (Personal communications 2007). These issues were highlighted in discussions and views around the national IAQ in England and Wales. At this point the influence of mental health advocacy should be covered in slightly more detail. Mature material concerns the intersection between mental, emotional and spiritual well-being.

2.1.4   Foci on International Mental Health Advocacy, National Networks and Schemes

Before a statutory mental health advocacy service had emerged in the UK, advocacy was taking root extensively in North America from the 1970s onward. Sim and Mackay (1997) were only slightly dated in their comparison with the UK situation when they stated that in

> …the USA the advocate is not only recognized in law and possesses rights of information access but all states are actually required to establish independent Advocacy agencies. As yet no such situation exists in the UK. Rather advocacy projects in the UK must rely upon the support and goodwill of local authorities, hospitals and community services to both support their existence and grant them co-operation. (Sim and Mackay 1997, p. 6)

Further international comparison (Forster 1998) showed that Austria and the Netherlands were viewed as having 'the two best institutionalised projects of professional advocacy in European mental health' (Forster 1998, p. 159). Both these programmes began in 1980. Whilst the Dutch programme relied on self-selection of patients, the Austrian selected them for being 'involuntary,' and therefore vulnerable. Dutch advocates were paid by the National Foundation for Patient Advocates, which guaranteed them independence from hospitals but meant that they did not benefit from contacts within institutions (Forster 1998; Klijnsma 1993). Instructed advocates in the UK may support clients to make complaints, but the former ICAS or PALS were more correctly parallel with American patient representatives, who, in a discussion of 'patient representatives' in the US in the 1960s, were also named 'health advocates' or 'ombudsmen,' as noted above (Ravich and Schmolka 1996). The emergence of mental health advocacy in other European and international contexts in relation to respective user movements would repay further study, but space does not allow (Carver. N and Morrison 2005; Dalton and Carlin 2002; Foskett et al. 2004a; Tudor 1996).

The sphere of mental health advocacy is closely allied to 'user empowerment' insofar as users in the UK are engaged, and therefore enabled to be, in control of their own destiny at the time of their mental disorder, which could involve detention in a psychiatric unit. This may be due to the pervasiveness of the voluntary sector in its support of user organisations, leading to a proliferation of mental health service-user groups.

In the UK, advocacy (including mental health advocacy) developed rapidly in the last 20 years of the twentieth century due to its status as a 'movement' and various associated groupings (networks and individual schemes) which sustain 'levels of enthusiasm and commitment found in few other fields of social endeavour' (Henderson and Pochin 2001, pp. 12, 14). Amongst important practice networks number Action for Advocacy (A4A). A4A was established as such in 2004, but originally founded in 2001 as Advocacy Across London, and regrettably folded in 2013 (Coyle 2013). One of its roles was in encouraging standards of uniformity through the Quality Performance Mark, which remains (Action-for-Advocacy 2006b, 2008).

There was also the National Advocacy Network (NAN), which organised conferences (NAN 2007), and the Older People's Advocacy Alliance (OPAAL), founded in 2002 and still active (Dunning and Joseph Rowntree 2005; Older-People's-Advocacy-Alliance 2008; P. Scourfield

2007; Wells 2007). But the longest standing network is the UK Advocacy Network (UKAN); based in Sheffield and founded in 1990 out of the activism of the Nottingham Advocacy Group (NAG),[2] it has been influential in the production of literature, including a Code of Practice for advocacy, which was cited in the earliest articles on advocacy practice. Its aims were displayed on its website:

> At the heart of UKAN is the belief that advocacy should be independent and led by people who have direct experience of using mental health services…
>
> UKAN promotes service user empowerment by representing issues from a user perspective in a number of national forums. It encourages the development of Patients Councils, User Forums and Advocacy Projects and offers information, training and support to both groups and individuals working towards mental health service user led approaches in any service. (UKAN 2006)

Beneath these networks there were 'many hundreds of small, local mental health advocacy schemes around the country' (see Henderson in Ryan et al. 2004, p. 206). This is a phenomenon which I consider as the expression of a social movement.

2.1.5   Understanding Advocacy as a Social Movement

Some exercises and research projects delineated the extent of the influence of advocacy initiatives (D. Barnes et al. 2000 [also cited in the NHS Mental Health National Service Framework chaps. 2 and 3]; Carver. N and Morrison 2005; Coyle 2008; Foley and Platzer 2007; Forbat and Atkinson 2005; McKeown et al. 2002; K. a. Newbigging and McKeown 2007).

---

[2]Newbigging et al. (2015) presented a detailed history of UK mental health user involvement. NAG organised the conference which spawned UKAN and consolidated support for patients' councils, issue-based and citizen advocacy in a militant-like atmosphere of workers 'downing tools' and on the march (Barnes and Gell in K. Newbigging et al. 2015, pp. 66–67).

Barnes et al. (2000) and McKeown et al. (2002) addressed forensic contexts, an area into which statutory advocacy services were expected to grow. Carver and Morrison (2005) and Forbat and Atkinson (2005) dealt with the local contexts of Scotland and Nottingham; Foley and Platzer (2007) covered the whole of London and concluded that existing mental health advocacy services operated in a climate of instability and uncertainty due to services provision faced with the specialist needs of a complex heterogeneous group (Foley and Platzer 2007, p. 632). This conclusion was elaborated upon by the findings of Newbigging and McKeown (2007) and then by A4A's summary qualitative study (Coyle 2008). Tew (2003) wrote that a different value base should include people as active participants or partners in their own recovery (Tew 2003, p. 24). In her account of user involvement, Wallcraft (2003) found at this time that BAME users were marginalised and needed their own network (Tew 2003; Wallcraft 2003, p. 29). However, there was a lack of an integrative, comprehensive study of advocacy practice, and in particular one which sought to illuminate and complete gaps with spiritual, cultural or theological dimensions in that practice. These were areas which were neglected but ones which have been recently recovered in IMCA to some extent.

To plug these aforementioned gaps would represent a refinement of advocacy practice, one of the aims of this book. Other connections between spirituality and advocacy practice were between the growing emphasis on a person-centred or spiritual approach and the theory and practice which was found in mental health advocacy. Other areas or modes of advocacy were influential and are at different stages of development—for example, advocacy for people with learning disabilities had a long history. On the other hand, advocacy for children, or for those involved in independent living projects, was relatively new and was being systematically tackled (Atkinson 1999; Parry et al. 2008; Payne and Pithouse 2006; Pithouse and Crowley 2007). As well as children, the involvement of patients (or 'service-users') in advocacy and research, the development of patient and public involvement (PPI) and later patient involvement in Health and Well-Being boards, were found to have features associated with personal, social and spiritual forms of advocacy.

2.1.6   The Literature of Well-Being and Spirituality in Nursing, Psychology and Chaplaincy

Thus the climate in which PPI and independent advocacy flourished, also characterised as a 'social movement of care' by Martin (2000), led to increasing concern in social policy with the issue of 'user involvement' and its problematisation. Studies on social work and users (Beresford 2007; Beresford et al. 2008; Croft and Beresford 1989, 1992), the critique of existing service provision which 'demands a voice in controlling standards and services themselves' (D. Ward and Mullender 1991, p. 21) and the lay, patient and consumer challenges to 'expert forms of knowledge and the authority of professionals' (Martin 2000, p. 1) were important in the development of advocacy. Criticism and complaint are two of the main ways in which those who use advocacy services are able to construct themselves and resist the system, and advocacy, often as mental health advocacy, gets involved with people at this point. The notion of 'emancipation' in mental health advocacy research was noted in a number of studies, for example, in the presentations offered by Tew (2003) and Wallcraft (2003), Fellow for Experts by Experience, NIMHE (National Initiative for Mental Health) and Senior Researcher—User Focused Research—Sainsbury Centre for Mental Health in the Social Perspectives Network (SPN) Study Day. Originally sponsored by the Training Organisation for the Personal Social Services (TOPPS England)- which later became Skills for Care-, and then by the Social Care Institute for Excellence (SCIE), SPN was a research network comprising users and non-users, open to a wide eclectic membership. (Bertram 2002; Cochrane 2003; Glynn 2003; Tew 2003, 2008; Wallcraft 2003). This indicated a need to explore empowerment at greater depth because of its link with the professionalisation of advocacy. Another area worthy of exploration in light of a development common with advocacy was that of spiritual care. This provided a link with Practical Theology.

The increasing printed and online material related voices from religion and spirituality to those from healthcare and mental health. Cornah (2006) conducted a literature survey on the impact of spirituality on mental health, and leading figures, Fulford and Gilbert, wrote and edited works on the importance of whole person and 'patient-centred' approaches in healthcare including spirituality and faith (See Cornah

2006; Cox et al. 2007; Coyte et al. 2008; Fulford et al. 1996; Gilbert and Nicholls 2003). This turn towards spirituality (hence, to some extent, theology) was evidenced in the growth of the special interest group in spirituality of the Royal School of Psychiatrists, which grew in membership to 1900 (RCPsych 2008) and was 2500 three years later (Powell 2011). This was also evident with the appearance of new journals, which connected (mental) healthcare and spirituality, such as *Mental Health Religion and Culture*. Here authors discussed issues such as prayer and well-being, and spirituality and mental health (Foskett 2004; Foskett et al. 2004a, b; Macmin and Foskett 2004; Maltby et al. 2008). Discussion of spirituality can unite practitioners who want to reflect theologically on advocacy and provide a platform for people of different beliefs to discuss approaches to healthcare, and the way in which that constitutes a conversation in Practical Theology has already been carefully framed. In this way it can be understood in the public square, say, by both those who are active in either healthcare or social care, and by religious pastoral care or chaplaincy professionals.

I commenced researching and writing on this topic in January 2007; since that time there has been considerable progress not only in the policy and practice surrounding advocacy, which I have indicated, but also in books and articles identified above, namely, aspects relating spirituality to healthcare and mental health. One innovation was the creation of the *International Journal of Culture and Mental Health* in 2008, and a number of important books. A leading figure was and is McSherry (McSherry et al. 2008; McSherry and Jamieson 2011; McSherry and Ross 2010), who has defended the role of nurses in extending the reach of spirituality as part of the therapeutic process in the National Health Service. He identified what he saw as the widespread willingness of nursing staff to engage in spiritual assessment and the need for further education in that area. The Royal College of Nursing Spirituality Survey, which was conducted online, had an extremely high (99 %) response rate.

This apprehension to engage with religious and spiritual aspects of care underlines the critical role education may play in preparing nurses to deal with religious and spiritual aspects of care (McSherry et al. 2008). Education can provide a safe environment in which to explore the relationships between personal belief and professional practice, and the boundaries that exist between patients and practitioners. (McSherry and Jamieson 2011, p. 1757)

Culliford (L Culliford and Powell 2006), a psychiatrist and active in the Royal College of Psychiatrists, produced a textbook noting that 'a satisfactory and accessible overview of healthy human psychology incorporating the spiritual dimension' was needful. He presented a 'new psycho-spiritual paradigm' and included an appendix on taking a spiritual history (L. Culliford 2010, pp. 9, 13).

The late and highly respected Prof. Peter Gilbert, active in NIMHE and, later, the National Spirituality and Mental Health Forum (Coyte et al. 2008; Gilbert 2007b, 2008, 2010; Gilbert and Nicholls 2003; Gilbert et al. 2006, cited above) continued writing and editing material. He 'brought together a stellar team of authors and produced as close to a comprehensive text on spirituality and mental health,' according to counsellor Tony Wright (Gilbert 2011; T. Wright 2011). A NIMHE Spirituality and Mental Health Project grew from a request made by Prof. Antony Sheehan to Peter Gilbert to make a creative response to the ramifications of the 9/11 tragedy in New York and in the wake of the bombings of 7/7/05 in central London. Gilbert (Gilbert et al. 2006, p. 15) linked the upsurge in spirituality after that, for example, inversely to a loss of meaning expressed in riots in France and to increased reference to spiritual issues in private sector management training.

Other British works included a collection of essays edited by Jewell and Kitwood (2011), 'Personality and personhood in dementia,' of use to spiritual carers (Jewell and Kitwood 2011). Karban provided an introduction to mental health social work in 'Social Work and Mental Health' (Karban 2011). From the USA, other edited collections aimed at professionals on the psychology of religion and spirituality in nursing were published; there was an emphasis on integrating spirituality and professionalism, evident from the titles chosen, for example, 'Spiritually integrated psychotherapy: understanding and addressing the sacred, ' by Pargament, asked how the therapist addressed the spiritual dimension in psychotherapy; he included the chapter title: 'In times of stress: spiritual coping to conserve the sacred…' (Pargament 2011, p. 4).

Reasons for the convergence and increased influence of spirituality-based texts include, firstly, the fact that many have their source in the USA, a more religiously-oriented culture with at least double the proportion of churchgoers than there are in Europe. However, greater transatlantic receptivity to this spiritual turn was evident in McSherry's work and the development of the British Association for the Study of Spirituality. Secondly, this imbalance may be due to the training expectation for chaplains in the USA where CPE is an integral part of ministerial training. (See 1.2 [above] and, for example, Aten et al. 2011; Barnum 2011; Karban 2011; P. Knight 2011; Pargament 2011; Peteet and D'Ambra 2011; Sperry 2012).

The role of IMHAs in assisting those caught up in the mental health system was crucial, or of IMCAs in portraying the views and preferences—including religious preferences—of individuals without specific capacities, contrasted with the medical 'best interests' decisions which healthcare professionals made. Both roles can be enhanced by considering ethical traditions and related course of action scenarios in more detail, as I showed elsewhere, and from absorbing aspects of the above works (Morgan 2011a). Some reflective practice takes place in current advocacy training but probably without detailed reference to philosophical or psychological stances. An increase in the cultural and spiritual understanding of individuals and communities could assist the performance of individual advocates and their organisations. This discipline could particularly be important with vulnerable adults and vital in relation to the Deprivation of Liberty measures, which the Code of Practice for the Mental Health Act 2007 set in train. In the light of this, in the next section I will consider the impetus for, and practical moves towards, professionalising advocacy services.

2.2   The Professionalisation of Advocacy

Given the status of advocacy as a 'work in progress' which was subject to many influences, part-social movement, part-profession, with the ambivalence which this entailed, it is necessary to position the discussion within the wider field of professional studies and to consider how to bring greater clarity.

Both Eraut (1994), who questioned whether professional knowledge was created by research or in practice (p. 41), and Schön, who discussed and was interrogated by Eraut regarding critical reflection upon practice (Eraut 2004; Schön 1983), provided formative material for this debate. Koehn (Koehn 1994) also related well to the topic on account of the broad approach to confidential boundaries and the 'good,' not least because of her examination of the trio of professions: medicine, the law and the clergy, with all of which advocacy is concerned, and this topic in particular (Thomason 1987, p. 5). For the purpose of comparing advocacy as an emerging profession with other professions at a more mature stage of development, literature on youth work and religious ministry, and on health promotion, which counted as professions at advanced stages, could repay study. But in this book I have used interviews from spiritual care coordinators who use advocacy skills to provide that comparison (Cribb and Duncan 2002; Dalrymple 2004; Eisikovits and Beker 2001; Emerson et al. 2000; Grover 2004; Rodwell 1996; P. Ward 1995).

How would further discussion of the theoretical basis of the professionalisation of advocacy look? Here is a practical example of how the intervention of one advocate was influential in the formation of legislation in the England and Wales High Court (Court of Protection). This strengthens an argument that advocacy's status is, to use a wildlife metaphor, now fully fledging.

2.2.1   Locating Advocacy Within the Professions

Independent advocacy needs arguably to advance beyond the perceptions often held by other professionals that advocates are only concerned with criticism and complaint and promoting a 'blame culture.' In relation to patient advocates, Ravich and Schmolka (1996) described the patient representative system and the Patient's Bill of Rights (1973) of the American Hospital Association as measures to redress effects of patient alienation due to a 'medical model' in the USA of the 1960s and 'increased emphasis on the treatment of specific organs, body parts or diseases instead of the "whole patient" and his or her psychosocial as well as physical needs' (Ravich and Schmolka 1996, p. 69). In advocacy practice some approaches based on a medical model were able to be challenged more powerfully than by social workers or NHS staff, or those individuals on their own. In 'Patient Advocacy' (1986), Ravich stated that alienation stemmed from the fact that large medical centres in the USA had, by that time, professional staff which had been divided into as many as 250 job classifications in 50 different occupational groups. In 1996, she added that the same centres exposed patients to as many as 65 different care givers in a single day 'at a time when they are most vulnerable' (Ravich and Schmolka 1996, p. 69). This pointed to the need for independent advocacy generally to support people with no one to negotiate complex health and social care systems. This seems to have been fulfilled with recent legislative changes outlined above.

Citing Johnson (1972), Eraut pointed out—in the light of this diversification—that the emergence of 'professions auxiliary to medicine' in Britain was due to the way in which physicians held sway in defining the scope of roles (such as that of the medical laboratory scientific officer), rather than representing the ability of each new occupation to be responsible for its own professionalisation (Eraut 1994, p. 3; T.J. Johnson 1972). Eraut highlighted the need for ethical codes to arbitrate between professionals and organisations, and the frustration of professionals with organisational procedures, and described the way the client- or person-centred approach had superseded the profession-centred approach because there were calls 'for the least powerful clients to be supported by "client advocacy"' (Eraut 1994). Professional advocacy has informal networks at best, but it also acquired the funding and ability to organise into a professional association with the support of (the former) A4A and its widely-known Advocacy Charter, an A3 size poster, and its Code of Practice and quality standards (Action-for-Advocacy 2002, 2006a, b).

2.2.2   Professionalisation and the IMCA Service

Eraut held a view of professions in terms of state-protected interconnected sets of power relations including service-users, service-providers and governments (Eraut 1994, pp. 3–5). Koehn (1994, p. 2) spoke of a professional ethic permitting doctors and clergy acting on behalf of 'clients who are unable to communicate their own wishes' (Koehn 1994, p. 9), a position which was close to those in receipt of non-instructed advocacy. In discussing the basis of professional authority she developed the concept of the moral, public pledge as a basis for authority. She spoke of a highly internalised sense of responsibility which was characteristic of professionals when they were dealing with vulnerable clients, and she related this to a number of definitions of the 'professional' (Koehn 1994, pp. 19, 55, 59), most notably linking the behaviour to public statements rather than a contract (from the Latin-based word: profession), a 'term applied to the public statement made by someone who sought to occupy a position of public trust' (p. 59).

In a critique of informed consent, she commented that, although designed to empower the client, it is predicated on non-involvement of the client who does not struggle to take charge of his own fate but is dependent on high responsiveness of the doctor to 'highly irresponsible client desires' (Koehn 1994, pp. 135–6). The introduction of the IMCA service was related to the 'sense of responsibility' after Koehn, for the IMCA Code of Practice stated that individual IMCAs must 'have integrity and a good character, and be able to act independently' (The-Lord-Chancellor 2007, p. 184). Secondly, in relation to the latter 'irresponsible client desires,' the UK MCA enshrined a new client-centred best interests' checklist, in which the role of the independent advocate (IMCA) was to ensure that the client was safeguarded. This means that a client who lacked capacity to make a certain decision was protected against her own judgement—for instance, she might wish to return to her own home, but the advocate would take a view which balanced her views and her own health and safety. This view may accord with that of the social worker but it may also differ from it. In this sense the notion of informed consent, which was the basis of standard instructed professional work, including advocacy, was displaced by the MCA and an advocacy-centred theory of best interests.

2.2.3   Capacity, Consent and 'Best Interests'

Luke et al. (2008) showed that clinicians thought that the IMCA service was 'largely impractical and unnecessary given current procedures for making medical decisions in patients' best interests.' However, clinicians also supported advocacy in discharge decisions by social workers because they believed that non-medically qualified advocates could make a valuable contribution. The study concluded that by holding these beliefs, 'clinicians are failing to have due regard for the IMCA service as a statutory measure for safeguarding patients' interests' (Luke et al. 2008).

These newly formulated 'best interests' were distinguished from what was previously known as medical-centred or care-centred best interests because they were firmly placed within the framework of the MCA principles which included independence from service-oriented decisions. It was also important to note that IMCA is a very specific but nevertheless non-standard form of advocacy. It was in the vanguard of the professionalisation of advocacy since it was a statutory provision which had been matured through the passage of the Mental Capacity Bill and then the Act itself, but the ethos of such a move had an impact on advocacy organisations since training to fulfil roles became not only statutory but an expectation by commissioners.

Dunn et al. (2007) noted that 'the MCA is consistent with the common law, but widens both the scope and procedures of a "best interests" determination to allow for a general model of substitute decision-making in everyday health and social care.' They argued that by decontextualising substitute decision-making, the MCA's procedures relating to 'best interests' may prove to be problematic, 'first, by failing to adequately resolve certain ethical dilemmas'—such as the need to assess a range of subjective evidence within an objective framework, balanced by a maximisation of personal welfare (p. 126); 'second, by reducing applied substitute decision-making to a series of compulsory generalised instructions; and, finally, by necessitating deliberation but offering little practical guidance to the process of determination' (Dunn et al. 2007). This demonstrated some of the complex material which advocates—in particular IMCAs—have to deal with.

Nonetheless, is creating the role of advocates unnecessarily adding to a plethora of health-related occupations, many of which are involved in supporting people without capacity to make decisions? These concerns will relate to SQ3 in Appendix 1 regarding advocacy's growth as an occupation and the use of public money to fund it. A consideration of the emergence of the occupation of the advocate has also included discussion of the nature of the training. This has been amongst the principle criteria by which advocacy may be claimed to be an emerging profession.

3   Speaking on Behalf of Another with Self-Sacrificing Vigour

An illustration of the growth of the concept of self-advocacy, which may also be partially true of mental health users and elderly users of both statutory and generic advocacy, was found in slogans from the user movement, which were employed in texts, and corresponding citation counts. A key text had the title, 'We can speak for ourselves' (P. Williams and Shoultz 1982)—and commanded 55 Google Scholar citations; another common slogan, 'nothing about us, without us,' was heard in an international conference in Eastern Europe and then repeated (in 1993) by leaders of Disabled People South Africa. Charlton's book, with the same title as the slogan drew 184 Google Scholar citations (Charlton 1998, p. 3). Sines drew attention to Williams and Shoultz's (1982) definition of advocacy as

...speaking or acting on behalf of oneself or another person on an issue, with self sacrificing vigour and vehemence. (Sines 1995)

This quotation and definition highlighted the campaigning, fervent, human rights-based or quasi-spiritual direction of advocacy, similar to the passionate expression of Wolfensberger regarding a self-sacrificial approach. It is this turn which I want to address more precisely in subsequent chapters of the book. Having drawn attention to the bank of literature which underlies the scheme, I have begun to face the key questions, Qs 1–3 (concerning a cross-disciplinary examination of the art of advocacy) and SQs1–5, by setting independent advocacy in social, political and contemporary professional context (Appendix 1).

I wished to draw attention to a number of other factors, which could be considered more fully, in order satisfactorily to construct a methodology to carry out qualitative research (Ely and Anzul 1991) in this area. There was 'grey' literature (specialist government reports, material produced by charities and study centres) and published journal articles, but very few in-depth studies of an increasingly important area. Many authors attested to evidence of a need for further research about advocacy (Doherty 2006; Gorczynska 2007; Mallik and Rafferty 2000; Sim and Mackay 1997; Xiaoyan and Yow-wu 2008). My title suggested a lack of 'theoretical resources' to carry out the roles of advocacy. These may be in the nature of training or of other professional expertise (Grover 2004; Reinders 2007).

To recapitulate, part of the aim of this book is to identify this lack by conversing with individuals involved as advocates or as clients of advocates, as carers of clients with advocates or as spiritual carers; to achieve this I analysed interviews using a case study approach (Beart et al. 2004; Helminiak 2006; Macmin and Foskett 2004; Strauss and Corbin 1998; Watt 1997). An online search showed that by narrowing down there were few substantial studies on independent advocacy and hardly any which attempt to relate independent advocacy directly to spirituality and theology. Yet literature from mental health and spirituality, as we have seen, indicated that this is an area of significant interest.

4 How Society Shows Its Respect for the Vulnerable

An IMCA provider involved in the Department of Health pilot projects stated that a particular advocacy service 'has the potential to become a key element in how society shows its respect for the autonomy, rights and protection of some of our most vulnerable citizens' ((DoH) 2008a). This assertion was made in the light of the funding flowing from the UK government through local authorities to the service. *A Right Result? Advocacy, Justice and Empowerment* was the title of an influential text in the practical study of generic advocacy (Henderson and Pochin 2001).

I have tried to show inherent tensions in debates about the history, nature, present and future conceptions of independent advocacy, and pointed to sources, internal and external to the actual discussion, which will inform the discourse. The aim of this book, therefore, is to synthesise appropriate spiritual and theological, sociological and philosophical resources in order to address a posited theoretical deficit in a practice. This attempted systematic review of definitions demonstrated a frustrating diversity in the sector which did not facilitate academic enquiry alone. The view of advocacy activists may well be that this is just as well because the academy is irrelevant to what advocates are about, and actually no theoretical unity can be achieved because certain minorities are ill-served on account of poorly conceived funding priorities. This was often more evident in public meetings and conferences than in the literature (Bowes and Sim 2006; Community-Services-Improvement-Partnership/London-Development-Council, 25-10-2007). For this reason the evaluation of interviews with advocates and others in the qualitative research component, which the review heralded, were crucial in how the story unfolded because they will build credibility and validity into the approach to the subject.

The history of UK advocacy could be understood as an independence movement being unduly influenced, for purists, by Department of Health funding, although the more recent austerity measures have put paid to this. The way in which a society becomes more human relates to voluntary and professional activities and how it conceives of both. My view is that evidence from the literature, and the testimony of the individuals involved in many aspects of the practice, shows that the underpinning theory, or the 'under-labouring'[3], is extensive and more important than to be left only to the advocacy sector. The well-being, humanity and spirituality of us all depends upon an enriched and enriching theory of advocacy. In the next two chapters I will provide a dialogue between the voices from the interviews which were undertaken and link them with those highlighted from a theoretical perspective.

---

[3]A term from Critical Realism.

4

Voices From the Inside—How Advocates See Their Occupation

The overall idea of an advocate is to be like an equaliser… (Sam)… a bit of a mouthpiece… (Janine)

1   Introduction

The next two chapters tell the stories of certain advocates whom I got to know and who also kindly agreed to be interviewed. The voices of the advocacy workforce are presented in creative conversation with those of service-users and with others who advocate in their own way. Of course, there is a personal element in my 'insider's account of the phenomenon' of advocacy since I explore culture intuited from one member's point of view (Silverman 2006, p. 102).

The Voices from the Inside will include those of Sam, who saw her role as promoting equity of treatment, as an 'equaliser,' or Janine (see subtitle), as an agent of communication, a 'mouthpiece.' Their chatter and insight will facilitate the formation of an occupational perspective including the pre-conditions, core conditions and essential qualities which characterise the emerging profession.

© The Author(s) 2017
G. Morgan, *Independent Advocacy and Spiritual Care*,
DOI 10.1057/978-1-137-53125-4_4

2   The Profession of the Independent Advocate

'Advocacy services becoming professionalised could end up being less helpful to service-users.' (Angela)

In the framework to his study on the academic development of medical students through time, Becker (1961) distinguished the notion of 'perspective' from attitudes, which I found a useful tool. The latter are unlike perspectives because they do not contain actions. Values are also dissimilar to them because they are situationally specific, the authors argued. Perspectives are…

> patterns of thought and action which have grown up in response to a specific set of institutional pressures and serve as a solution to the problem those pressures create… [They] are related directly to dilemmas faced by the persons who hold them. (Becker 1961, p. 36)

I look at the perspective of independent advocacy practice as pressures grew around its pragmatic existence. Unlike medical training, formal requirements for the training of advocates are still at early stages. However, the culture of advocacy stretches back in time (Chap. 3), is richly textured and contains within it certain understandings which challenge how it may be sustained. In addition, there were debates at A4A events (including the National IMCA Conferences) about whether advocates should be registered by bodies such as the Health Professions Council. Opinion was divided evenly, or slightly biased against, whether this was a good idea. It was thought both that such a registration could compromise independence and, alternatively, that such a step was probably inevitable due to the statutory acceptance of IMCA and IMHA (Personal Communications 2008–2011).

In the following account, advocates outline reflections upon the culture, identity and activities of practitioners in relation to an emergent profession. To form a picture of the emergent culture, I listen to the voices of all participants and intend to show by what the emerging professional identity is framed and influenced.

2.1   Primary Professional Perspective: Tacit Knowledge and Common Sense

'There are certain qualities that you need which are just not trainable' (Ruth)

In the period 2005–2010 independent advocacy underwent significant changes, with the IMCA and IMHA services coming on stream, and the 'primary group perspective' of advocates was seen in a certain light. From her mental health advocate perspective, Ruth argued that 'there are certain qualities… which are just not trainable.' She continued:

> *Sometimes it's the right thing to do (without training) and sometimes it will lead to problems in terms of stepping out of role…* (Ruth 2007, November 21)

This related back to the essential value placed on independence and the sense that any professional competence should be premised on an aptitude measured by the experience of the service. Alongside this lay a definite empathy with the service-user and a suspicion of professionalism: this circumscription of 'role' was defining of the professional advocate. Ruth's views will be revisited.

With the landmark introduction of statutory advocacy from 2007, service-led expectations about training were altered, and so I also take account of how this perspective changed. In this phase I concentrate on the how rather than the what, for example, how they were equipped, and later I will consider the nature of the qualities which they required. An underlying aim was to look at views on advocacy training and how that may be enhanced. Was there a weight of evidence that participants would place more value on individual character rather than on role, on informal rather than formal learning and qualifications, and on expressed values rather than rigidly-tested competencies? In short, I asked whether there was a leaning towards tacit knowledge as a means of achieving credibility with advocacy. I take this to mean the use of transferable skills by someone less than expert to perform a competent function (Eraut 2004).

I found that 'common sense' was a useful theme in pondering informal learning, for example, in Cornwell's (1984) account of health and illness in London. Giddens conceded that common sense was more than 'cookery-book knowledge' and that it derived both from experts such as priests, magicians, scientists and philosophers as well as in part from the 'accumulated wisdom of laypeople.' But Giddens also identified the problem of how this composite 'stock of knowledge,' observed by Cornwell, could then be interrogated by sociological method. Cornwell described the way in which the status accorded to doctors affected the information he got from participants as a 'process of interaction between the medical and common-sense approaches in which the medical approach is usually, but not always, dominant' (Cornwell 1984, p. 22). One of his interview participants compared the work of the medical and social work professions:

> They've had to learn something to do their sort of job. Social workers, nine times out of ten anyone could do it…. he knows what he's talking about… a social worker, I think it's just a job anyone can do, anyone with common-sense. (Cornwell 1984, p. 183)

This showed a gradation of status based on the possession of tangible qualifications and how a common-sense approach is rated lower. However, an alternative view upholds its value in what laypeople or 'users' also have to offer as their critical 'common sense.' This may include the 'oil' of the social worker, which smoothes the operation of the system. The dilemma is at the heart of advocacy and of this particular enquiry, as I show in the second half of this chapter.

2.2   Establishing Professionalism from Experience

Turning to the participants, whose voices and perspectives I embed in the narrative, I introduced Kevin (See Appendix 2) and alluded to the professional and personal motivations driving him. Unlike many others, he did not mention that he had been a volunteer before earning a living in the sector. Kevin did not want to define advocacy too precisely:

> *Advocacy is something done by people called advocates, (and there are) people who are not called advocates but are paid in different roles. I think in all things*

it is better to think in terms of overlap, with responsibilities within a contin-uum. (Kevin 2008, January 14)

The unwillingness to specify the nature of a paid role, although the refer-ence is definitely to roles which are paid, shows either confidence and flexibility or an over-optimistically broad understanding about how indi-viduals will be able to understand what they need to do to support and represent clients. Kevin has been supporting people in different roles throughout his life and is now in a management role. Here he speaks about the qualities he would look for in a new recruit:

some quite deeply personal things here, and I think some… can be trained and developed, but I certainly tend to look a lot more for the skills people have and their ability to present well and to think things through rather than rigid knowledge based competencies… (Kevin 2008, January 14)

When Kevin stated that there are *'things that can be trained and devel-oped…,'* the implication is that advocacy is 'caught not taught,' but what normative framework can provide clarity on what can be trained and developed? Relying only on skills could undermine the wish of leaders of advocacy services in the voluntary sector to be taken increasingly seriously by commissioners. In the next section I look further at the evidence from practitioners about the basis for the view of advocacy as a profession.

Ruth was a participant with a long experience in advocacy. She spoke about how she had joined a large organisation with a good reputation and had access to quality short courses. This, she thought, prepared her for advocacy work, but she said, nonetheless, that she did not think *'good training makes a good advocate… (but) the most important thing about an advocate is their attitude… and there's no training for that.'* Ruth did not feel you can *'train people'* in empathy although she felt you can *'channel people's qualities and skills and hone them and develop them.'* She felt that there are advocates who passionately want to perform a role but had no access to training and who could therefore have a poor experience of advocacy because they would have problems *'stepping out of role'* (Ruth 2007, November 21).

Ruth's view of training was that she had experienced some good quality courses but also that their variability stemmed from being needs-led rather than qualification-based. She did not state this explicitly. She also pinpointed the ambivalence of advocacy training I referred to above and the tension between a common sense-based or passionate attachment to the practice, which leads to justifiable action. On the other hand, that action could be detrimental to the image of advocacy and, more importantly, for the client if the advocate did not know what they were doing. Ruth did not, however, present training as the answer. On the contrary, when Ruth advocated 'attitude' and said that *there are certain qualities you need which are just not trainable,'* this seemed to evoke high standards which it would be unusual to require in other professions without recourse to formal training. If one did not say of a brilliant medical student that she cannot become a doctor on account of a deficient attitude, then one ought to do so.

Nebi, another advocate with a long record of service and from a different organisation, also placed emphasis on 'attitude.' He said that the most important thing is attitude because *'you can learn the knowledge, you can learn the skills'* but *'if you are the kind of person who is not going to listen and will try to control people you will not be a good advocate'* (Nebi 2007, October 22).

2.3   Attitude, Common Sense, Training and Independence as Pre-Conditions

From the weight of evidence and experience, I learnt that the role of the advocate is strongly independent. Having reviewed perspectives and a range of voices, I will now focus on this sense of independent identity, which depends so much on attitude, and on the area of training. But how does one account for 'attitude' in the context of professionalisation? It is an area that is difficult to quantify and therefore to measure. To start with, Nebi felt that *not* listening and controlling others are *not* endearing qualities and are likely to disqualify an aspiring advocate (Nebi 2007, October 22). Olive also made a parallel point when speaking of her work facilitating a self-advocacy group (see Morgan 2015 for details). She said that it was *'difficult not to take over a controlled group, you've kind of not got to be a control freak...'* (Olive 2007, November 7).

Being open and listening is an attitude which, Ruth argued, it is not possible to train. Janine offered (below) a full description of the actions which constituted a training process and contributed to a primary professional perspective. She spoke of training experienced as *'hitting the ground running'* (Janine 2007, October 1). Fauzia also inferred that training is something you *'pick... up as you go along'* (Fauzia 2007, October 1) and felt it was an important role which should be attributed with a recognised title. It was for her, as a BAME individual and migrant, something that by practice she recognised because *'before I came here I didn't even know advocacy exists (but) I knew it worked'* although she had always supported or helped people (Fauzia 2007, October 1). So for Fauzia, a volunteer who stumbled upon advocacy, the emergence of the profession was empowering in that it provided in the first place a professional niche she did not know existed. Both attitudes and training contain variables, but elements of progress in skill development were also evident in reports.

For a number of participants, training was synonymous with 'ongoing learning' rather than an award gained prior to employment, and it had constituted no more than the induction after they were first employed in an organisation. Janine explained how scared she was when she was first employed as an advocate and how she grew in independence. She also reflected on her experience as she picked up the role of an advocate as being *'scary'* and making her *'nervous,'* for Janine needed to read for herself and learn about the MHA and mental health tribunals, how to interpret client files and the database, and to be self-motivating regarding administration. The use of role plays featured in her training, which she *'hated.'* In fact, it seems from the description of the induction that the addition of drama skills could also be helpful, even if a bit daunting:

> *You would shadow another colleague and so you would watch them fulfilling their role, and then role plays... and then being shadowed by a colleague... taking on the role <u>independently</u>, um, sort of being seen doing the job.* (Janine 2007, October 1)

This example of ongoing learning from Janine in mental health advocacy indicated an emphasis on practice rather than formal education. Although 'attitude' may not be trained, it seemed possible that attitude may be modelled. This apprenticeship approach (as in medical or teacher education) with dry-run scenarios (as in the role plays which were mentioned) was alluded to by other participants. It is widely used in advocacy organisations and represented a process formative of occupational, if not professional, independence. Ruth also compared what is required in mental health advocacy with different qualities which should be borne in mind as the outcome of training and which are needed in community care or non-instructed advocacy:

> *Mental health advocacy has some more challenges and conflicts than some other advocacy areas… actually you have to be quite sharp and acute to realize what is actually patronising and disabling and what is empowering. I think you also have a sense of what's risky to the client, you have to have a sense of what's erm… you have to have* <u>common sense</u> *actually. I think you also need to be quite reflective… you need to be able to stand back and check what is happening between you and the client, and your relationship with that client.* (Ruth 2007, November 21)

Ruth warned against being 'patronising and disabling' when working in a client's best interests and spoke for the need to be empowering. In explaining this, she said advocates should use advanced skills when dealing with clients who may be severely disabled or who lack capacity to make their own decisions; they should also have some knowledge of, or training in, risk assessment ('*sense of what's risky to the client.*'). This begs the question of how these skills would be assessably imparted. The appeal to 'common sense' represented a summary of what she felt was important in advocates in the pre-conditions for their engagement in practice and importantly in building rapport, or 'empathy,' with the client. Ruth has been clear that training alone cannot provide these. I will now examine these pre-conditions in the wider range of advocacy.

Bella (see Appendix 2) was an experienced advocate and advocate trainer who had been involved in advocacy with people with learning disabilities during almost the whole of its lifespan. She stated how advocacy is a difficult craft and how complex an independent professional perspective could be. Her repetition of 'not easy' established this as a theme:

> B: *I don't think advocacy's easy, I've got to be honest, it took me a year to 18 months. When I started working for [name of organisation] to truly get to grips with it, and I learnt a lot from the volunteers.* (A. Norah and Bella 2009, December 14)

I drew conclusions from participants from different branches of advocacy, whether they were working with people who are able to communicate verbally or with those who communicate non-verbally, or very little. Firstly, the skills required for advocates to carry out their independent roles are diverse, discreet and particular to client groups, and may need instructed or non-instructed approaches. Secondly, the participants themselves indicated that the advocacy role is not one which is easily comprehended and that some people do not have the aptitude to make it in the profession. However, ironically the level (level 2/3)—as it stood in 2010—of formal qualification required to be an advocate made it difficult to claim that the occupation was a profession. As Angela reported in 2007, training depended on which organisation advocates worked for and on the '*mixed bag of training*' they sampled. As advocates moved from one organisation to another, consistency suffered, so from the point of view of a mental health advocacy organisation, '*a consistent and coherent package of training*' was definitely called for, she felt (Angela 2007, October 1).

In desiring such a training package, Angela reported that later her own organisation did provide cultural awareness training. Angela also said that '*if people were approaching things with an empathetic, sensitive and common-sense approach, while you might not have in-depth cultural awareness, you might have sympathy and empathy to engage with them to be able to establish what they needed*' (Angela 2007, October 1).

One dictionary definition of 'empathy' is the 'power of projecting one's personality into, and so fully understanding, the object of contemplation' (Little et al. 1983). Angela mentioned that while she would hope that people would be empathetic, it was not guaranteed. Her words suggested that advocates would be able to use research skills (based on the tacit knowledge mentioned above) to discover what they needed to know, an approach to advocacy training which I found typical with other advocates. Changes have been gradually implemented in relation to national and commissioning expectations about statutory IMCA and IMHA training. These were discussed above (1.6.4) and assessed now by annual reports and more recent articles and books, which cover their implications ((DoH) 2013; Dept-of-Health 2010b; Luke et al. 2008; Morgan 2011a; Newbigging et al. 2012; K. Newbigging et al. 2015). In relation to Angela's views, it may be possible to argue that any role, including that of the advocate, required individuals to be aware of their training needs. The question is what evidence there was to show that a formal prescriptive training requirement will produce practitioners of a higher standard than currently prevail. The generalists with degrees and backgrounds in other disciplines, who, sometimes combined with other careers, populated statutory advocacy, may be as qualified for their role, albeit by a different means, as social workers are for theirs.

When I considered a different form of advocacy, that is citizen (or volunteer) advocacy with people with learning disabilities, some of the views of Norah and Bella were consistent with the establishment of a professional perspective. As we will see below, the background against which these two participants contributed was as champions of volunteer-based advocacy, the form which has a large claim to be independent. Bella was a citizen, or volunteer, advocate and Norah was a coordinator of volunteers. The original principle of volunteer advocacy was that all that should be funded (rather than advocates themselves in paid roles) was an 'advocacy office,' which was supposed to resource volunteers. Bella informed me that she was influenced by Wolfensberger, acclaimed as a founder of citizen advocacy, and this position was argued for polemically by him:

> We make the assumption that societies will be better societies if their individual members voluntarily take care of each other.... In contrast to either not taking care of the needy at all, or mostly doing it impersonally, indirectly, distantly, involuntarily, or on a ***paid basis***. (my italics) (Wolfensberger 1995, p. 21)

When Norah and Bella were asked about the qualifications which they thought should be held by advocates, Norah replied,

> *Oh, well we always used to say that <u>common sense</u> was the main priority to have, but then you have a certain amount of intelligence or be able to speak if you are going to speak on someone's behalf…* (A. Norah and Bella 2009, December 14)

When Norah cited 'common sense' as a requirement for advocates, she appeared to link this desired specification with an established history. Elsewhere Norah showed a profound knowledge of some leading figures in citizen advocacy, John O'Brien and Wolf Wolfensberger. For Norah, the main motivation in advocacy was focused on a relationship with a client, or, in Wolfensberger's terms, a 'protégé' (or what we may now term a 'mentee'), as we will see below. The theme of common sense seemed to be associated with a world where volunteering was highly valued, namely, the field of citizen advocacy. Wolfensberger was himself disparaging of one definition of 'self-advocacy' because he felt that it did not account for the reality of disability:

> It is important to distinguish between authentic citizen advocacy, and other advocacies that are positive – e.g. Scandinavian Ombudsman – and harmful degradations – e.g. self-advocacy that denies the merit of other forms, and denies an actual impairment. (Yeadon 1990, p. 3)
>
> The advocate's loyalty is to his protégé, not to an agency or even the advocacy office. Thus, he is a volunteer to the person, not the agency… (Wolfensberger 1972, p. 221, 1995)

Wolfensberger drew attention to the notion of the ombudsman—standing for trusted and fair representation—which indicated the frequent and necessary association of the advocacy role with an 'auditing process' in the administration of care services and by extension with complaint-making. Interestingly he evoked a competition for recognition between different forms of advocacy in its early history. But the precepts about loyalty to the individual and the place of voluntary activity were also exemplified by Norah and Bella:

N: That's the reason the whole movement came about, that we're independent of it, we're not paid
  B: Yeah
  N: ... so we won't lose our job whatever we do...
  B: ... I don't feel that if I make a decision and support someone in a certain way that I'm going to lose my job... I've got to be honest if the choice came between following [name of organisation] party line and doing the best I could for the person, I'm going to go for the person. (A. Norah and Bella 2009, December 14)

I wanted to show in previous sections that for clients with mild or moderate learning disabilities, self-advocacy represented a stage in achieving greater independence, gaining a new voice and increased choice. The demanding axioms, which Wolfensberger set out, were optimistic in relation to human nature and financial costs, since volunteerism was at their heart. They shaped the primary independent perspective which many advocates share and with which, moreover, they have been imbued historically through inhabiting organisations in which his ideas have matured. The pressures which Wolfensberger reacted to from the 1970s onwards may in some ways differ from now, but the campaigning rigour he demonstrated has been deeply formative.

Moving on now from a general consideration of what it means to be an advocate, which emerged from conversations and reading literature, and having proposed a primary professional perspective of advocates, in the next section I will focus on professionalisation in advocacy as perceived by advocates themselves. I will begin by listening to the voices of clients or self-advocates, and to those of the comparator profession of chaplains/spiritual care coordinators. Through these lenses I will scrutinise—in a more synthetic manner—the origin of advocacy in a 'movement' and how its characterisation by resistance to professionalisation could have affected its trajectory. As part of the argument I will consider SQs 2 and 3 (See Appendix 1) regarding different views on professionalisation across advocacy and the financial value which advocacy can bring. I noted that a 'perspective' was, after Becker (1961), a 'pattern of thoughts and actions' which had grown up in response to institutional pressures and in relation to the dilemmas which are experienced in action by those practitioners. Their perceptions were that training in itself, as they experienced it, did not directly produce practice. It was rather about developing innate qualities along the way. I found that pre-conditions to be an advocate involved a certain attitude and a willingness to learn from a varied and flexible approach in training. This primary professional perspective was based on the practitioners' own possibly lower expectation of training at that time since mandatory training for statutory advocacy had only just arisen. The perspective also included, through the evidence from Norah and Bella and others, a rooted commitment to the individual, which is based on the consciousness that advocacy is at its heart an independent, voluntary activity.

2.4   Combining Vocational and Practical Perspectives

> 'We need to be able to show that (our) services... are better to spend money on than other things that are often done by social care' (Kevin)

In considering the status of the 'emergent' profession, it was important to hear what advocates said, but always to set this consideration in the centre of what clients or service-users thought about the role. The impact and outcome of the actions which advocates take can be measured by the views of clients, usually the best metric for the valuation of a service. This issue also related to SQ3, which represents a strand in the argument, showing the rising service-user movement within health and social care. SQ3—advocacy's value for money—is where I launch out below.

2.4.1   Self-Advocates' Views on the Value of Advocacy

Members of a self-advocacy group—Louise, Michael, Pixy, Germaine and Whitney—who were in that sense advocacy clients, were asked about whether they thought being an advocate was a proper job.

> (Co-f = Co-facilitator)
> Co-f: Do you think being an advocate's a proper job, do you think it's a proper job like your support worker, or like a lawyer, or
> Pixy: [name of borough] council

Co-f: Yes, like someone at [name of borough] council who helps you with housing; do you think it's a proper job…
Pixy: Yes
Co-f: or do you think it's a nice thing that people do?
Germaine: Yeah, it's a proper job
Whitney: It's a proper job
Pixy: Proper job
Whitney: You get paid as well
(Louise et al. 2007, November 23)

Some self-advocate service-users, such as Pixy and Germaine, who were both involved in NHS committees, namely 'Partnership Boards'[1] (as service-users) and Whitney, who had experience of being supported in a house-move, thought being an advocate ranked alongside other professionals who supported them in their lives. In a section from another interview, when asked if being an advocate was like a job, organisation, a political party or a movement, clients responded:

(F. = Facilitator [the researcher]):
Mary: It's a job
Madonna: Take people who have learning disabilities on special holidays…
F: So it's a job but it's an enjoyable job because you get to go on holiday with people
Barry: … I think more than 1 person is involved…
F: Yeah, it's collective, more than individuals
Barry: It's more than a job, it's like an organisation, like [name of organisation], someone's got to start it off. (Micky et al. 2008, May 14)

The service-user Barry asserted that advocacy appeared to be *'more than a job… like an organisation.'* As a carer for his partner, he showed an understanding that the administration and organisation of a workforce, or 'organising people,' was a central element of the emergence of the occu-

---

[1] 'When the *Valuing People* White Paper was published in 2001, it established local Learning Disability Partnership Boards as part of its delivery mechanism. Partnership Boards were set up to bring together all the relevant local agencies and stakeholders, and to give a voice to people with learning disabilities and their family carers,' wrote Minister Phil Hope ((DoH) 2009, p. 4) .

pation as a professional service. This insight was built on by advocates. The interview schedule included a question about whether participants felt that advocacy was a movement, service or profession. Deliberately open-ended, it illustrated an emergent professional perspective amongst practitioners, subject to the raised expectations following the introduction of statutory advocacy services in 2007.

2.4.2   Advocates' Views on Advocacy as a Vocation

I begin with a side-light thrown out upon the discussion and recall the desirable emphasis on volunteering which Wolfensberger (see (c), above) commended. The journey, from volunteer to professional paid advocates, was reflected upon by spiritual care coordinators Sarah and Karim, who saw advocacy as *'more professional than a movement'* (Sarah) but characterised by being more *'practical'* than chaplaincy, and although she was not sure how to write up its *'professional requirements,'* she felt it was also *'vocational.'* Karim was more eloquent about the nature of this vocation.

> K: *I think it's a vocation of people… who have come out of an institution and feel they want to give something back. Perhaps they start by being given a small task and if they feel they are helping, I think they genuinely feel they want to help. The ones that I have met are certainly like that…* (Sarah and Karim 2008, December 4)

It is worth noting that participants in a qualified or parallel professional path, that is, that of the chaplain, saw the movement dimension as a threat (see further Dorothy, Chap. 5, Sect. 5.2), or as detracting from professionalism. Origination as a movement, in contrast, constituted a strength within advocacy, as Maria and Janine show further below. In her assessment from a limited experience, Sarah associated advocacy firstly with notions of practicality and then with professionalism and vocationalism. This ordering is significant since it accords broadly with how advocate participants viewed their practice. From Karim's riposte, he focused on the benefit for the clients of mental health advocates, who succeed by giving something back from what they have gained from their own experience. He thus appeared to modify Sarah's assessment by moving the element of 'vocation' higher up the ladder. That is to say, the formation of vocation is determined to some extent by personal lived experiences, a feature which participants (e.g. Angela) have emphasised. The practical 'user-focus' has been mentioned above (3.2.) and will be examined further in 5.4 via a chaplaincy-based consideration of the 'use of self.' This reality of the user-focus has affected the development of the status of the profession in the advantages and disadvantages of volunteer and/ or user involvement, which will be discussed further below. As for formal professionalisation, I have already described the way that employment in certain advocacy roles requires NVQ Level 3/4 certification and that there is a possible move towards registration by the Health Professions Council or some other body, for some or all advocates into the medium term future.

Angela, furthermore, described how the evolution into a profession is taking place, in her view, by making parallels with other disciplines such as those of the occupational therapist or counsellor...

> It...has... changed from a movement to being a service, and it's now in the stage of being a service but becoming professionalised, similar to other disciplines working in the mental health community... (Angela 2007, October 1)

However, she was quick to highlight what she viewed as the advantages and drawbacks of the developments:

> I have mixed feelings about it; I think from the point of view of service users receiving a coherent and structured service there are benefits to advocacy being a service; but I think that in the process of advocacy becoming a service there is a danger that the essence of advocacy is lost, and by the essence I mean the advocate identifying very strongly with the service user and engaging with the service user on their own terms. By the advocacy services becoming professionalised there is a danger that they just become like any other statutory service. They could end up being less helpful to service users and more concerned with their professional status than with the needs of service users. (Angela 2007, October 1)

This point again could be linked with the implication from Karim's observation that a vocational strength could be lost. Maria pointed out that there has always been the view in *favour of making it more professional* based on an assumption that potential service-users would be alienated from volunteering to do advocacy if they had to attain a professional qualification. Although it could seem like it carried more weight, Maria said, at the same time, becoming part of a *'multi-disciplinary team'* could weaken the purpose of advocacy:

> ... *I think the idea that advocates are not coming from a qualified area... makes it unique, and what makes advocates extremely approachable to service users...*

Maria maintained that for peer or citizen advocates who have been active a long time in advocacy, *'the idea of formalizing it is a bit scary.'* In addition, smaller advocacy groups fear they could be *'swallowed up by bigger advocacy groups who are more professional.'* This would also result in a loss of the 'local' emphasis since *'most peer advocates have been in hospital, have been a patient, (and) know it first-hand...'* She also therefore wondered about the outcomes if one were to do a survey enquiring whether users preferred advocates to be qualified or not (Maria 2007, October 1).

Building up independent advocacy as a service meant increased contact-time with clients but quality could be sacrificed to quantity, Angela seemed to suggest, where quality resided in the relationship with the *'service user on their own terms.'* Maria mentioned the *'approachability'* of advocates as a unique selling point for peer and volunteer advocacy. She also suggested that non-professionalism may be attractive to some mental health clients in that they are thus able to identify with advocates if they have been service-users themselves and are 'local,' and that those who know the system 'first-hand' may find the need for a qualification off-putting. It is possible that the focus on the client which was at the root of the movement may be lost if qualification-attainment is a primary goal in training.

The qualification issue has been addressed by setting the qualification low—at level 3—although in practice many advocates have degrees or other professional qualifications. The level also ensured the occupation remained an attainable objective for a non-graduate. However there may be a danger that the setting of a 'low bar' would be seen as patronising to the ambitious mental health service-user, for example, who wished to advance in the occupation in order to move into another profession. In relation to the maintenance of professional standards and capacity, it has proved true that larger less costly advocacy groups dominated the market when the transfer of IMCA advocates (under TUPE[2] legislation) took place from one service provider to another for reasons of cost efficiencies. With the most self-sacrificing advocate (who is prepared to work harder for less reward) this could benefit the client. In reality it could mean that advocates who have been achieving high standards in one service are prevented from doing the same in a different service because they are forced to increase client lists, prompting a similar crisis to that affecting social work teams in times of austerity. They may then leave the occupation of advocacy (perhaps for social work or the psychology service) through dissatisfaction because their continuing professional training needs are not met and if they can as easily be employed in a related field. This possibility of attrition (which was borne out by my experience) was an example of how the market and economic conditions may have undermined a valuable emergent profession.

2.4.3   Moral Resistance to 'Professionalisation' and Wardrobe Tips

In this next section I compile some evidence to show how answers to Q3 regarding cultural or spiritual approaches to questions of professionalisation may be attempted. Above I spoke about how Reconstructed Empowerment (RE) may be a way of addressing the question, and below I will acknowledge that the theme of resistance to aspects of professionalism and corporate identity may be useful in this regard.

Reactions to the piecemeal approaches to advocacy training were shown from the accounts of varied participants, in particular from that of Janine. She also shared her thoughts on new approaches to training, but firstly described how she felt advocacy existed on a continuum from a 'movement' to 'professionalisation,' via the status of 'service,' and said she felt that *a bit of me won't catch myself... considering it as a professional status.'* Janine foresaw accreditation and qualification (in October 2007)

---

[2] Transfer of Undertakings and Protection of Employment legislation in the UK.

as *'new measures'* on the horizon and that the movement would *'trip'* to a service, but at that point in time she viewed it clearly as a *'service of information and support'* (Janine 2007, October 1). This notion of resistance was also echoed in a more emotive way by Sam:

> *how you dress is really important, like wearing a tie is a very bad idea when you are working as an advocate because you don't want to be just another suit, because they get loads of those and they are generally people who don't do what they want them to…* (Sam 2008, February 13)

Sam's wardrobe tips merged attitude and appearance apart from qualifications. As a longstanding advocate she situated advocacy and fed prospectively into a secondary perspective. Nebi also had a developed perspective on advocacy seeing it as *'an extension of the civil rights movement'* with the benefits of professionalisation seen as clear *'structures and boundaries'* (Nebi 2007, October 22). Following his caveats about attitude (noted above) he continued in interview to praise circumspectly the on-the-job training, or learning style, employed in the light of new professional expectations, for *'it allows you to reflect and to practice, to move forward by identifying gaps in your learning. So I would say it's a good way if you become more experienced…'* Nebi felt advocates would need to *'get up to speed with the legal issues… and sometimes the attitude as well.'*

> *I would say it is good to have this ongoing training identified as people are performing; and there should be a minimum amount of training as people without it cannot be an advocate.* (Nebi 2007, October 22)

However, Nebi prefaced this realistic appraisal with more qualified views about the emergence of the profession from a movement:

> *There should be a balance between the enthusiasm and the coordinating of the movement; and the campaign of the militants, but again with some rigour and principles and guidelines that are ascribed to professions. But we should look at… service users. Peer advocacy, for example would not like the advocacy movement to be hijacked by certain types of principles, qualifications… in terms of making it more open to people who were or still are a victim of institutions.* (Nebi 2007, October 22)

Nebi's contribution, set alongside those of Maria and Angela above, highlighted the enduring prominence of the user and volunteer advocate focus, with a vocational emphasis, without which a move towards pure professionalisation could be compromised. In speaking of *'victims of institutions,'* Nebi referenced de-institutionalisation or the movement to community care (in learning disability or mental health) as we will find Peter regarded safeguarding in 3.2.6, below. Nebi's terminology also highlighted how safeguarding is now a central commissioning responsibility for statutory advocacy, but Nebi was mainly concerned to secure the place of peer advocates in the emerging profession. He sensed that those who have been discriminated against in the care system could empathise and support those who are still in this situation. This is seen as a feature of RE.

Both Angela and Janine (above) spoke chronologically in October 2007 when the IMCA (and certainly not the IMHA) services, which would later affect mental health advocacy, had not been fully implemented. Since then, a more consistent approach to advocacy training was being introduced by a range of providers certified by the Department of Health. With its gradual introduction there was at the time a shrug of resignation that it was inevitable, some advocates questioning it as a barren exercise. On the other hand, the involvement of advocates in safeguarding procedures had imposed the need for an element of statutory training. This affected the most recent perspective on the profession of advocacy in irresistible ways. Overall there was a sense of the practice developing a more professional ethos with a dash of deconstruction of what it means to be professional. This was connected with the independent focus, and yet there needed to be consistency and agreement to establish a reconstruction. Professional expectations from government were also more recently very much to the fore (Department-of-Health 2013; Legislation.gov.uk 2014; Newbigging et al. 2012). I would like RE to exemplify an approach paralleled in the spiritual care professional role, and for this to contribute to a more culturally and spiritually adept stance in advocacy.

Sam said later in the interview that she has had *'limitless amounts of training... but I think basic advocacy is quite simple and should be'* (Sam 2008, February 13). I will explore how *'simple advocacy'* took fuller shape as it developed and the views of practitioners in this regard, and later indeed how this simplicity also acquired fuller dimensions in 'Deep Advocacy.'

2.5   Primary Professional Perspective as 'Movement,' 'Service' or 'Public Pledge'?

Does the role and occupation of the advocate reside any longer in a movement, or is it a service now? (SQ3) This question also pertained to the area covered in Q1 and 2 and related to the debates within advocacy schemes about professionalisation (SQ2). Evidence from professional advocates was predominantly that it consisted in a service because, as Peter stated, (it) *'doesn't feel like a movement at all, it feels like a service...,'* (Peter 2008, December 9, l.85). The costs of prolonging it as a volunteer movement were considered prohibitive:

> P: *I think, look it's an option, volunteer advocacy, um, I suppose our observation at [name of organisation] is it's not an obvious saving, you know volunteers need support and training... but it's not necessarily the cheaper option or one which provides better advocacy to more people. I think research would need to demonstrate that really. I'm not sure there is an advantage in attracting more volunteers, and we'd be spending more money on getting individuals volunteering. Getting more volunteers doesn't feel like it's very important to explore particularly in the professionalisation of the service...* (Peter 2008, December 9)

The economics of advocacy were influential, and as Kevin, in future-proofing mode put it, there was a need to show commissioners not only that one service is more cost-effective than another but ultimately that advocacy is *'better to spend money on than other things that are often done by social care'* (Kevin 2008, January 14). I will show in Chap. 5 that there are benefits in the deployment of volunteer mental health advocates who are service-users. In addition, the link between contemporary advocacy with its origins as a new social movement, as I delineated, was borne out by some other evidence from advocates, as we have seen, and crystallised by the participant below:

Well, it is a movement, it is a movement... but I don't think though you have to be part of the movement to be an advocate and to provide a good service. It's a service movement. (Laughter) It's a professional service movement (Laughter) Oh god, I think you can alienate good advocates by focusing only on the movement aspect; you can alienate strategists and decision makers in society also, but if you don't hold on to the fact that it has been and continues to be a movement then you can get swallowed up by the system so it's about balance, isn't it, and ultimately it's about clients. So it has to be a service. (Ruth 2007, November 21)

Ruth's observation usefully encapsulated an emerging recognition of the increasing status of the occupation in the changes which it has undergone in its journey—definitely as a service—moving towards that of a profession. Together with this, Ruth demonstrated a degree of happy confusion about the status, which is emblematic of the attitude or tone which practising advocates take and of the way in which they regard their role. Kevin spoke above about the *'overlap'* with other services and the idea that advocacy took place within a *'continuum.'* Peter furthermore warned against making a special case of advocacy:

It's about service provision to people, it's about providing a service in a particular role alongside other services which have specific roles and responsibilities so I am not precious about it... being something special. (Peter 2008, December 9)

The self-effacing approach shown by advocates is in keeping with the person-centred and user-led focus which predominated in the sector. Let me summarise how the professional perspective is to be seen from the evidence of those with whom I engaged.

So far in this chapter I have considered the emerging profession of independent advocacy and the public good. I indicated how the initial perspective in advocacy practice was harnessed to the principle training requirements for statutory advocates. Training requirements were applied more generally to all those employed as advocates and specifically by their provider organisations with various degrees of pressure. Units 301–304 of the basic IAQ included respectively 'Purpose and Principles of Independent Advocacy—Skills, Knowledge and Competence,' 'Providing

Independent Advocacy Support,' 'Maintaining the Independent Advocacy Relationship' and 'Responding to the Advocacy Needs of different groups of people.' Rather than a top-down competency-based or university accredited qualification, the IAQ represented a City and Guilds Level 3/4 vocational standard. This was arguably a flexible instrument and could capture some of the advantages of activities- and attitudes-based criteria in the deployment of advocates as well as point to a framework for further professional development. Participants, including advocates, and a few users of advocacy skills, for example, chaplains, reflected upon the development of the occupation into a profession.

As I listened to the voices of advocates and clients, I considered the emerging profession from the point of view of training, attitude and experience. I presented a 'primary perspective,' which consisted of a perception that advocacy was an independent, voluntary activity which was generally remunerated; within this framework training was acquired informally but was not rated as highly as certain innate qualities which may make someone a 'good advocate' such as 'common sense.' Building upon this, in (d), I noted an increased preoccupation or inward gaze (perhaps influenced by the step-change in 2007 to a statutory and therefore more contextually 'professional' service), which from the evidence meant a more realistic and positive attitude to training. This emergent perspective was also distinguished by a wish to balance the heritage of advocacy as a volunteer movement against the pressure of commissioners upon providers to demonstrate 'value for money.' The heritage of advocacy as a movement was important and remained so. One way of understanding this phenomenon, which I introduce at this point, would be to assign the label of 'prefiguration' or 'prefigurative politics' to the trajectory I have observed.[3] This analysis may be helpful as it is consonant with a Practical Theological vision within a Critical Realist framework, and because it is democratically rooted and capable of denoting the owned and recon-

---

[3] I was grateful to Mick McKeown for this commentary at an advocacy conference (private conversation at Community-Services-Improvement-Partnership/London-Development-Council, 25-10-2007). McKeown et al. (2010) pointed out that 'prefiguration (after Gramsci et al. 1972) describes the way people in social movements try to practise what they preach in trialling their ideals of alternatives in the actual mechanisms of transition. They have a vision for a future world, and, in the act of trying to realise it, they try to model what they are trying to achieve. This is about the ends of achieving a new social order being as important as the means' (McKeown et al. 2010, p. 36).

structed ideology of advocacy, travelling through a continuum from a movement to some kind of service.

Despite the above, the new perspective viewed advocacy predominantly as a service rather than a movement. Within that there were increasingly professional characteristics defining the activity of independent advocacy. These included reference to an optional Advocacy Charter and Quality Performance Mark provided by the London-based A4A, mentioned above in Chap. 1 (Action-for-Advocacy 2002, 2006b, 2008a). But these developments together fell short of an arrangement whereby independent practitioners would form part of a professional association bound by a Code of Practice or would be accepted as part of a health or social services professional council. Nevertheless the MCA Code of Practice does impose unity on one form of advocate, the IMCA.

I also discussed the relationship between specialist IMCA advocacy and professionalisation. There I cited Koehn (1994). Koehn, a Professor of Ethics, used the triad of professions—medical, legal and Christian religious ministry—in order to posit her models of professionalisation, for example, with a section on 'salvation' (Koehn 1994, p. 104); this was perhaps more usual in an American rather than a UK philosophical context, in which my book is located. But the spiritual and theological domain was also particularly relevant in the interviews I conducted. Koehn brought out a definition of a profession as

> an occupation for which the necessary preliminary training is intellectual in character, involving knowledge and to some extent learning, as distinguished from mere skill; which is pursued largely for others, and not merely for one's own self; and in which the financial return is not the accepted measure of success. (Brandeis and Poole cited in Koehn 1994, p. 19)

Insofar as the emergent perspective in advocacy recognised the importance of induction and values (attitudes) in practice, it was evident from participants that although the emphasis was on experience, there was also a need for knowledge and some learning. This knowledge, which was based on a theoretical deficit, as I argue in this book, increased—at least as a perception—with the advent of statutory services and the refreshed realisation of, and pressure on, the place of advocacy services after 2007, especially in terms of IMCA and IMHA. In this way advocacy needed to review, assert and possibly improve skills, knowledge and learning. In this emergent professional perspective, it also held true that the occupation was not pursued 'merely for one's own self' and that financial return was negligible. There was nevertheless evidence of a healthy scepticism of the advantages of a purely professional service and fear of losing the expertise of service-users or volunteers. This could be characterised as an ambivalent turn-toward-professionalisation.

In her rejection of expertise alone as a ground for professionalism, and likewise of client contracts, and in advancing 'the public pledge' or 'covenant'—a Judaeo-Christian concept which also brings in theology to a point—as the ground of professional authority, Koehn modified her original definition of a professional as:

> An agent who freely makes a public promise to serve persons (e.g. the sick) who are distinguished by a specific desire for a particular good (e.g. health) and who have come into the presence of the professional with or on the expectation that the professional will promote that particular good. (Koehn 1994, p. 59)

Koehn added that the 'expectation' existed that a professional will provide a certain good because sometimes people are brought by others into the presence on the strength of the pledge such as people in a coma or the mentally disturbed (Koehn 1994, p. 190, footnote 4). In addition to the arguments she utilised for her professional ethical framework, Koehn's views were pertinent to the overall message of the book and in particular to the lens of *virtue ethics* through which, I argue, theoretical benefit for advocacy practice can be seen. This helped to provide a theological model by which to assess advocacy practice and contributes to the overall argument via response to Qs 2 and 3. I have considered the perspectives which advocates brought to their practice in relation to its status as an occupation turning into a profession.

In Sect. 2 of this chapter I turn more precisely—using emergent analytical categories—to consider those attitudes, activities and actions which constituted the role as it became a more professionalised service.

3   The Essence of Advocacy Culture: Reconstructed Empowerment and Action Based on Equality

The essence of advocacy… (is)… identifying very strongly with the service user (Angela)

My focus in this second section is driven by what advocates think they are doing in the roles which they variously fulfil and how that shapes their practice in a more direct than theoretical way. This relates practice more tightly with the lived experience of advocates and embraces the advocacy experience of those who are not employed as advocates; the section is situated in the argument in response to Q2. So in this section I listen largely to the voices of those involved in formal advocacy and also to some extent to those engaged in a distinctive advocacy role, in this case spiritual care coordinators or chaplains, in order to provide comparisons and contrasts. I will also give some attention to the views of clients, but not as much as I will in Chap. 5.

I will begin to develop models to describe what advocacy roles consist in by looking at the nature and qualities of the advocate. Arguing in this and following chapters that advocacy demonstrates a vital, altruistic, moral or spiritual attitude to powerlessness, from themes drawn from interview data I will utilise the term 'Reconstructed Empowerment.' In relation to this, the label 'Action Based on Equality' will describe the cluster of themes referring to actions which, over and above attitudes, augment the professional perspective common to advocates. Both Reconstructed Empowerment and Action Based on Equality are refinements from categories which grew out of the qualitative information gained in interviews. In the next section I will show how Reconstructed Empowerment and Action Based on Equality emerged from the views of participants as part of the conceptual analysis. These themes will thus become tools to cultivate the material which I was offered.

From here I concentrate on the essence of advocacy, the core qualities which make advocacy practice effective and the context in which advocacy services happen. In the following sections, some quotations are extended in order to give full voice and depth of personality to the characters; I will also use 'live' quotations to introduce sections (as I have with the 'essence of advocacy,' above), link the argument in the spirit of creative conversation and thus produce a tableau vivant effect.

3.1 Support, Empowerment, Trust and Other Core Conditions

I say, 'No, it's not about me, it's about you…' – Janine

From the evidence gathered, I found that for independent advocacy to have outcomes, certain pre-conditions (attitude, training, independence and common sense, for a start) needed to be present. In addition, I discovered other more subtle categories from my conversations are helpful—namely, the ability to *'think around corners'* for a service-user who at some point is not strong enough to do that for herself (Kevin) or being prepared to *'go around the houses'* by giving extra support but taking care with emotional boundaries (Janine). So what do detailed soundings from advocates about their roles indicate, and how do they build the case for the professionalisation of advocacy? Firstly, I will consider a mini-example of one advocate's view of her role. Janine reflected on the role and the technical functions of both an instructed and a non-instructed advocate:

> … *Um… the role of an advocate…um… there's a saying you know… helping people to express what they need, what they feel is lacking in terms of their care and treatment… I sometimes refer to myself as, be it clients or professionals, as a bit of a mouthpiece because I am literally repeating back what clients have asked for support with.* (Janine 2007, October 1)

As well as the delicate framing of support, the theme of power was raised by Janine. I will deal with this elsewhere regarding the way it was used by other participants (e.g. Dorothy, 5.2), and explicitly the 'expressed powerlessness' of advocates. However, the use of power, as we shall see, is not straightforward because there is a discrete power which advocates exercise and which the descriptor 'reconstructed empowerment' encapsulates (See further in 5.1 *'We don't have any power but we can empower'* (Jana)). So Janine reflected on the deployment of influence to get alongside clients:

So there's a honesty when working with clients because you don't want to set up a kind of false hope, again I can't tell people, you know... 'I can't promise you any outcomes, all I can do, is convey what it is you feel you need, or is likely your concern is, I can never tell you what you're going to get,' but if you don't ask you don't get, and so yeah, being realistic, honest, being patient... (Janine 2007, October 1)

It was therefore around the provision of a service, based on the liberality or charity of the individuals rendering it, who may be religiously or humanistically motivated, that advocacy, named as such, was centred. This was the culture which I investigated. However, that culture was also deeply dependent on the needs and rights of individuals being supported, with the consequent exercise of human moral or spiritual will, public service and the common good. This correlation of new and ancient forms can enrich the theory of advocacy. Whatever was done, whether voluntary or paid, it called for reflection, analysis and new applications because in their intention advocacy services were based around the needs of the most vulnerable people who either could not express themselves or had difficulty doing so. The nature of disabilities led to marginalisation, invisibility and unacknowledged and uncharted areas of vulnerability. Placing the individual at the centre was a slogan of the financial personalisation movement in the NHS and social services in England. But a truly personalised approach would also be holistic, integrated, related to that which is done voluntarily and not ignorant of, but prepared to embrace, the cultural, spiritual and transcendental insofar as that was capable of being present or evoked in every individual or community. How could all this then be personified in the advocate?

3.2   Essential Qualities in Independent Advocacy

The order in which the qualities are listed requires comment: they are actually a range of carefully pursued characteristics, drawn from the interviews which I conducted with my participants. They can therefore be classed as essential qualities in the formation of the independent identity of the advocate. Elsewhere, in training material or other qualitative studies, similar sets have been produced, which may bear comparison with those which follow.

Comparably, Rai-Atkins (2002) listed, for example, key aspects of 'culturally specific advocates, identified by BAME service-users, services and carers as:

- Someone you can talk to in your chosen language
- Someone who listens and understands your issues and experience
- Someone who has the authority to challenge professionals
- Someone you can identify with, that is, through culture, identity and gender
- Someone who can offer consistent long-term support
- Someone you feel you can trust
- Someone who can provide accurate information relevant to individual needs
- Someone whose services are accessible at a community level'

(Rai-Atkins 2002, p. 36)

This section absolutely relates to Qs 1 and 2 in setting out the moral and spiritual basis of Practical Theological take on this emerging profession. The qualities described here were also developed from the thematic analysis I initially used in relation to the gathering of this data. I will principally use the explanation building approach to amplify the voices of participants as I describe the nature of these qualities. The first four subsection themes are ordered according to the frequency of their occurrence in my interview data. Subsects. 3.2.5–7, although drawn from the key questions, are more theoretical in their provenance because they relate to what statutory independent advocates are bound to do, and also they lead into the next stage of the argument in the chapter.

3.2.1 Ability to Listen

Listening to clients, as counsellors are aware, is not a straightforward skill, as Angela pointed out in stating that listening and allowing individuals to make their own decisions were priorities for advocates: *I think many people actually struggle with the second one, in fact many people struggle with both of them'* (Angela 2007, October 1). Angela drew attention to the fine balance between attending to clients and allowing them to make their own decisions, which is particularly relevant in non-instructed advocacy where best interests principles allow for the taking of unwise decisions. Jana, Janine and Nebi also explained how attentive listening is incumbent upon advocates in their support of clients:

> J: *I think being able to listen, that's the most (important), and keeping calm; I think if you have got these two you can make a good advocate, with extra training and things like that, but I think you have to be a good listener, and be calm at all times...* (Jana 2007, October 22)

Asked about the most important quality for an advocate to have, Janine replied that it was *'listening skills.'* She said often a lot of information needed *'filtering out'* but *'in between somewhere there could be an issue...'* (Janine 2007, October 1). This point was developed by Nebi:

> *I think the most important thing is the attitude of the advocate in working with the people who are to, or potentially who can have a say in their treatment, and not to... control them... an advocate has to be an excellent communicator, a good listener to people when they are having difficult times and also a good negotiator...* (Nebi 2007, October 22)

Janine spoke of the need to read between the lines of what is being said: this is true in instructed advocacy and perhaps more so in non-instructed IMCA practice (defined in Chap. 1) when clients lack capacity to make decisions, and the role of the advocate is to discern what individuals may wish for under the radar of their being deemed medically or socially to lack capacity. We have previously heard Nebi speaking of the priority of the advocate's attitude over, say, knowledge of mental health law. Here he argued for the use of social and pastoral skills in ensuring that clients get fair treatment in *'difficult times.'* Bella contributed insights from her work with people with learning disabilities:

> B: *When I'm training citizen advocates we do an exercise about the qualities that are essential to an advocate and, as Norah says, the one that I like to high-*

light, the most important one, is the ability to listen… I think that is one of the most important ones, and not everyone can. They think they can but they don't do it very well. (A Norah and Bella 2009, December 14)

Bella observed accurately that listening well is underrated and hard to achieve. Bella also said how she is very choosy about those whom she trains. Sam gave more shape to the skill of listening carefully to those with disabilities and being mindful of what advocacy is. She recommended working *'positively with people with disabilities'* by concentrating as much on *'what they can do, as on what they can't do…'* Being a *'good listener,'* picking up information in *'different ways'* and *'having a degree of mental organisation'* were important as well as keeping in *'mind at all times what the principles underlying advocacy are…'* Sam also mentioned that qualities of patience and good communication are intrinsic to the occupation of the advocate. This meant you must *'have a sensitivity to how people communicate differently,'* according to Sam, and be patient, open-minded and *'allow clients to function at their own pace, and not, as far as is possible, attempt to operate at your pace'* (Sam 2008, February 13).

3.2.2 Showing Patience and Communication Skills

Patience and communication skills (bearing in mind that communication was evoked as a core condition) were also qualities which other participants raised as crucial in practice, for example, Fauzia with mental health clients and Olive with individuals with learning disabilities:

You have to be approachable, understanding, you have to be able to communicate, sometimes it takes a long time to understand what people want so you have to have a bit of patience, you have to be caring, there are a lot things which you have to be. (Fauzia 2007, October 1)

So I think you have to be able to listen to people, and to communicate with people in a way that encourages their dialogue. You have to be very patient and let people talk about an issue, talk round an issue, talk 'til the real important things come to the top. (Olive 2007, November 7)

Olive also said that much of the work she did was group work and that this required a group to support each other, and *'you have got to be able to facilitate the group so that everyone in the group has an equal chance to communicate'* (Olive 2007, November 7). Fauzia's perceptions were similar to those of Nebi in emphasising a caring approach; Janine similarly commended a listening ear (as we have seen above regarding attitude) and being tolerant of people's stories even if they are irrelevant to the issue the advocate has to deal with. Olive was even more conscious of this need for pastoral sensitivity as she spoke about facilitating group dynamics in self-advocacy with people with learning disabilities so that people had an equal opportunity to contribute in order to support each other and develop communication skills. Fauzia had also mentioned the ability to communicate as had Nebi (above); Ruth had some views on these aptitudes as well, as did Sam, who stated that *'you need to be a confident speaker and communicator'* (Sam 2008, February 13):

> *You need really good communication skills, you need to be able to deal with conflict on a daily basis, erm without losing your temper, erm, and also to always to keep in mind what it is you are getting for the client so you have to alter the client focus...* (Ruth 2007, November 21)

Sam's comment was related to professional behaviour, and Ruth usefully linked communication skills to conflict resolution and the need to be focused at all times on the client. This characteristic I could describe as typical, in that the advocate takes the side of the client in seeking to achieve her wishes; and it is thus possible to draw out further skills and specific styles through which this takes place, in negotiation, for example.

3.2.3   Negotiation Skills and Tenacity

Earlier in her interview Ruth spoke of the underrated competences needed by advocates in the actions they take; she did not *'think people recognize the difficulties and challenges of being an advocate.'* Ruth stressed empathy, the need to have *'an ability to see it from (the) position'* of the clients and *'a knowledge base of what it is that they are up against.'* Ruth said she did not think there is any *'point in you having an understanding or empathy if you don't actually have any idea how to help that person at all, you don't know the systems or negotiating.'* She felt you should be really skilled and knowledgeable about the context you are working in (Ruth 2007, November 21).

Here Ruth emphasised the need for empathy (seeing it from the other's point of view), but she also stressed the need to know the system, to possess the negotiating skills in order to take action on behalf of the client in an intelligent way defined by a knowledge base. But, as Janine indicated, in restating the realistic restriction in what advocates can do, or any power they may hold, much would depend on the ability to anticipate the negotiation activity which the client may require.

> *I suppose sometimes you want… to negotiate a bit more for a client but if you haven't preprepared that, then you can't really go there because you have got to talk to the client about what they want you to do. So there are times when it feels actually very limiting, what you can do to help somebody.* (Janine 2007, October 1)

Again this action derived from the voluntary or enforced powerlessness; Janine noted the lack of clinical training, which related back to the previous discussion about perspectives, and the need to prepare in order to influence professionals regarding clients using negotiation skills. The manner in which this influence was exercised is shown by a conjunction of other moods, firstly from Maria, then from Ruth and Sam:

> *Um… enthusiasm, some empathy, and focus, um, and oh, determination, I suppose, that someone has their views heard.* (Maria 2007, October 1)

Ruth said that the practitioner had to try hard to *'remain an advocate,'* which would involve not being a *'cold fish'* but *'multi-tasking.'* She envisaged someone who would *'challenge and be quite robust when the system comes down… not just… on the client but the advocate.'* Saying no, *'being persistent and dogged to ensure that issues are dealt with'* were also desirable in the view of Ruth (Ruth 2007, November 21). This was elaborated on by Sam:

And you have to be tenacious, you have to be able to deal with situations where people are against you and still be able to behave professionally. And you have to be able to carry on nagging at people, and not give up. (Sam 2008, February 13)

Determination, doggedness or *'nagging'* and tenacity were cited as qualities which advocates feel they need to have in their armoury. In her contribution Ruth drew attention to the challenges to the 'system' which independent advocates are involved in and one which IMCAs, for example, are statutorily able to carry out if they disagree with a decision. Ensuring that issues were dealt with for an individual as part of the *'robust'* work, where no one is necessarily on your side, is an area in which advocates specialise. There are two more clusters of qualities and actions by which advocates may be recognised: firstly, participants expanded on the basic definition of advocacy as 'speaking up.'

3.2.4   Enabling Quieter Voices to Be Heard

Ruth (Sect. 2.3) described the advocate's role as *'standing alongside'* and *'helping people's voices to be heard'* individually and socially, by which Ruth meant that there are political implications to the role: she saw advocacy as supporting an 'arm's length' challenge of the system as it impinged upon clients (Ruth 2007, November 21). Maria has already amplified this stance, above, in describing the *'determination… that someone has their views heard,'* but this is clarified further when she was asked about the tasks of an advocate:

Um, I guess it's in terms of… the main one is ensuring that the client is able to raise their issues in the way they want to, in the appropriate way… and for that an advocate needs to be, to have an awareness of the culture, and the system to be able appropriately, to be able to inform the client. (Maria 2007, October 1)

This perception regarding the tasks of the advocate is built on by Fauzia in answer to the same question:

Providing information, that is the biggest thing, people don't know what information they want, so clarifying that, and, again, advocating for people, supporting people, speaking on their behalf... quite a lot of people can't really express their needs, often on ward rounds people need help, so it feels really rewarding when you get someone's point of view across. (Fauzia 2007, October 1)

Fauzia drew attention to the engagement (which she valued) in meeting the diversity of needs of people whose first language may not be English and who are, as we shall see later, doubly or triply disadvantaged perhaps on account of stigma. They did not know about the support that they could get nor were they able to express themselves. Again, in Maria's contribution, I identified a stress on learning a culture and actively confronting what in this case was probably as much a mental health system issue as part of an equal rights agenda. An example of this will follow in the next section. Countering disability or addressing 'hard to reach' groups were issues which Sam (as we will see) also mentioned as she cited the need to ensure everyone has...

an equal say, that they are able to express themselves and have access to their rights as though they didn't have a disability or whatever it is that defines the client group. Um, and I think there are several parts to that: I think the most important part of advocacy has to be supporting the person to speak up for themselves and to have as much control for themselves as is possible. (Sam 2008, February 13)

Enabling a client to be in control was a vital factor in the empowering process which advocates are engaged in as part of their activity, in which the client defined the form and extent of that control. Even when the client lacks capacity to make certain decisions in non-instructed advocacy, the theory of the MCA 2005 attributes a benefit of the doubt to an individual, for example, in maximising their capacity or allowing an unwise decision to be made. I continue this section with some remarks from advocates regarding the integrity of the advocate.

3.2.5   Deploying Integrity and Good Character

Although it is a specialist form of advocacy, the MCA 2005 Code of Practice determined that IMCA advocates should have integrity:

> Advocates (IMCAs) must 'have integrity and a good character.' (Dept.-for-Constitutional-Affairs 2006b, p. 184)

This basically meant that they need to have satisfactory enhanced Criminal Record Bureau checks. It was instructive, however, of the essence of advocacy that some examples from participants backed up this requirement. In line with the special role which Fauzia occupied (above), she has already spoken of the need for the individual advocate to be *'approachable'* as has Maria (see b (ii)). Olive described the dynamics of supporting a self-advocacy group as dependent upon trust:

> *I think it's important that people, the members, or the people that you are working with, trust you. You have to be able to build relationships with people very quickly, otherwise people are not going to tell you anything, and then your role is redundant.* (Olive 2007, November 7)

The attitude demonstrated by Olive meant that work with people with mild to moderate learning disabilities, according to her, was done on their behalf and there are no decisions taken without them; as she says, quoting the advocacy adage, *'nothing without them'* (Olive 2007, November 7). In discussing the recruitment of advocates to his organisation Kevin deliberated on the choice, as we saw above:

> *I guess the key question I always come back to is, 'Is this person somebody whom I would want myself, or somebody I was close to if they needed an advocate?'... and it's... about whether that person inspires that trust and competence or confidence.* (Kevin 2008, January 14)

The choice which Kevin related to perceived trustworthiness or integrity may seem subjective. But in setting out the essence of advocacy and for the activity which advocates undertake, I have also demonstrated that such qualities and actions cohere with the expression of advocacy in a certain group of practitioners.

3.2.6 Statutory and Non-Statutory Safeguarding Role: '*It's About Trying to Protect People*' (Peter)

At the crux of advocacy was also the notion of 'safeguarding,' which Kevin and Peter emphasised. Although it had been formalised in the IMCA role in that decision-makers are able to make referrals to IMCA advocates in safeguarding (vulnerable) adults procedures, these circumstances have always been a reason for involving generic advocates. Kevin went on to define the role in adult protection or safeguarding:

> *It's about decision making so it's about people having support to make decisions and it is also — and I think we have almost come full circle in this — because it is also about safeguarding people, about protection which I think some of the early perceptions of citizen advocacy really emphasised really strongly, protecting the rights of people who would otherwise have a really raw deal. I think as, yeah, as language has changed, and as thinking has changed, it really sounds embarrassing but I think we have returned to it particularly with the IMCA role.* (Kevin 2008, January 14)

Kevin also said that '*early perceptions of citizen advocacy*' held safeguarding in high regard and that we had therefore come '*full circle*' (Kevin 2008, January 14). But later in the conversation, as we saw above, Kevin affirmed the specificity of the practice of advocacy in saying that

> *if we keep it very nebulous and say it's what anyone and everyone can do there is no real difference then we lose some of the important safeguards and quality that you can have in a service but that you can't have in the things that I choose to do for my neighbour.* (Kevin 2008, January 14)

The passion which motivated early expressions of citizen advocacy was evoked by Kevin, along with the realism that this intensity may not always result in the effective social service which advocacy was intended to enable. A similar enthusiasm, tinged by sober acceptance, was again elicited from Peter when questioned about his motivation:

> *What encourages me about it... a lot of the work is protective, not letting bad things happen rather than supporting really good things happening... and that varies between local authorities and time and place. A lot of the work is trying to resist some bad things happening to people... it is about trying to protect people, to protect people from service changes, political mantra, saving money, really just to protect people... These days it really is about trying to help people to hold onto what they've got... and it is about accountability of the local authorities and the PCTs so that they are challenged... then it's about the confidence to challenge them...* (Peter 2008, December 9)

Peter highlighted the preventative role of safeguarding practice in the general experience of the advocate and showed how the role not only fitted in with what other professionals did but also provided that monitoring function in relation to the social worker, for instance, as he performed as an employee of the local authority. Defined by laws such as the MCA or the MHA, certain independent advocates, such as IMCAs and IMHAs, were thus in a stronger position to safeguard vulnerable individuals, on account of their independence from the statutory services.

In regard to its professional identity, my evidence shows that advocacy has undergone an evolution over the last 30 years, from a movement to a service and that it is *'at the stage of evolving into a profession,'* according to Angela (Angela 2007, October 1). Her feelings about this development were mixed, as we will see further below. She felt that the transformation of advocacy into a service would mean that its essence—which could be that which one chose to do for one's neighbour—could be lost:

> *By the essence I mean the advocate identifying very strongly with the service user and engaging with the service user on their own terms.* (Angela 2007, October 1)

This would have an impact on the relationship with commissioners who are responsible for the sustaining of advocacy but who are not focused on classic advocacy, that is, interested in whether individuals volunteer to do things for their neighbours or not. In that sense I asked her if statutory advocacy in the voluntary sector may provide a bulwark for this classic advocacy; and later Angela clarified why the increasing involvement of the third sector in providing mainstream or statutory services may not achieve this:

> … *I think advocacy organisations should do far more to engage with statutory service providers to enable them to understand the role of advocacy better than they do. I think advocacy services often shy away from engaging with statutory providers, that's a mistake really. Advocates need to be able to explain what their role is, the limits of their role, the boundaries, then they will be able to gain respect, advocacy providers find it easy to blame statutory providers for not understanding their role, many advocacy providers don't engage with statutory providers appropriately.* (Angela 2007, October 1)

When I asked her if this was because sometimes nurses or social workers saw themselves as advocates (see Chap. 1) or because social work managers referred to team members as 'advocates,' Angela replied:

> *Where it is properly explained to them my experience is that the nursing staff have really got it and have pulled in advocacy services…* (Angela 2007, October 1)

This, however, may be otherwise with social workers or NHS staff in other London boroughs from the ones which Angela has experienced.

3.2.7   Loving One's Neighbour as Oneself—*'To Be Like an Equaliser' (Sam)*:

So far in this section I have argued that concerns, stemming from a close identification with the service-user, to seek justice and to promote equality from an independent point of view, to safeguard individual rights and the need to go beyond what one is able to do for one's neighbour in terms of a commissioned provision (as Kevin argued) were intrinsic to the motivation of advocates. I will now turn to data from different sources in which participants gave their views on what qualities are required in practising advocates, which may have these sorts of outcomes.

Sam related the role and qualities of the advocate to an agenda of equal rights by saying that he had dwelt much on the notion of advocacy and that the role involved being *'like an equalizer'* and to try to work with (people and) support them to the extent that they have *'access to their rights as though they didn't have a disability or whatever it is that defines the client group'* (Sam 2008, February 13). Different types of responses (from spiritual care coordinators and clients) threw further light on the nature of the practice. I will go into further detail on these responses in Chap. 5. Norman, a chaplain, echoed this particular function when he spoke about *'levelling out the imbalances of power'* (Norman and Colin 2008, September 11).

Bella described the process of seeing a client move on as *'problem solving'* and that it gave her *'a terrific buzz'* when the client felt *'totally confident in disagreeing'* because that meant that they saw the relationship as *'a totally equal partnership,'* which also counted as a *'compliment'* (A. Norah and Bella 2009, December 14). What may be an emergence of an element of capacity and new expression of personality could be counted as action which has resulted in equality and empowerment for the client. Secondly, the points of view of two service-users, Whitney and Pixy, members of the self-advocacy group Help Advocacy Reach Town Heath (HEARTH), confirmed a client image of the advocate as one who listens, befriends, communicates and accompanies.

(Co-f = Co-facilitator):

F: ... What sort of person is an advocate? What is an advocate or what should an advocate be like?

W: Someone like Pamela... she... she... I remember her, she is my key-worker... talk about things, our relationship, our families, I know all about it

Co-f: Pixy, what sort of person do you think an advocate needs to be? If you are going to be a good advocate, what sort of person are you?

Pixy: Nice, polite... decent, speaking polite, and also it's very important to listen to you. And speak up, try to learn a bit more, and like... coming to your meetings, it's important to go to, to go to partnership board... you need more and more meetings. I've done three years as a rep, and I'm taking over (from) Nigel...

(Louise et al. 2007, November 23)

4   Conclusion

In Chap. 3 I constructed a history of advocacy related to mental health nursing and expressions of advocacy in other countries and related this also to PPI, the user movement, self-advocacy and recent health and social care legislation. This narrative mapped on to the key questions (Qs and Q1 to a large extent) and most of the SQs at various points. These were voices from advocacy history and policy formation. Building on that, in this chapter I facilitated a critical conversation between the voices above and those of practising advocates. Thus, in Sect. 2 of this chapter, when considering the emergence of advocacy from the professional and training perspective, and subsequently turning to the culture of advocacy in Sect. 3, I related respectively to Q1 and Q2, and presented the voices, experiences and perceptions of advocates regarding their own formation and practice, based on the above expectations, and by including chaplains using advocacy skills within the conversation. In this way the essence of advocacy practice and activity began to be defined normatively through correlation with spiritual and theological themes from the influences of chaplains.

5

Voices From the Outside—How Non-Advocates View Advocacy and How Advocates Address Social, Cultural and Spiritual Needs

people need friends, people need colleagues, people like us, it's so good, I'm powerful… (Pixy)

1   Introduction

From inside the world of advocacy, in this chapter I change the focus to how independent advocacy is seen by those external to it. I concentrate particularly on the perceptions of spiritual care professionals and their views of independent advocacy (Q2). Therefore I am discussing the question of the emergence of professional advocacy consciously within the disciplinary context of Practical Theology. This relates also to Q3, as well as to other SQs (Appendix 1). According to the argument, by listening to the voices from clients and from another quasi-independent profession (e.g. chaplains), as they reflect on the method of independent advocacy, it will be possible critically to correlate the voices and build the argument that spirituality, theology and advocacy theory are mutually enriching.

© The Author(s) 2017   **135**
G. Morgan, *Independent Advocacy and Spiritual Care*,
DOI 10.1057/978-1-137-53125-4_5

2   Independence, Power, Virtue and Spiritual Support

'We don't have any power but we can empower.' (Janine)

In two of the interviews I conducted, Olive, a self-advocacy group coordinator, and Bernard, a chaplain, used advocacy skills to support users in their encounters. In so doing they shaped a 'virtue ethic' through the empowerment of the other in complex systems. Bernard wished to push the boundaries of his role to advocate for a patient in the NHS, and Olive felt that *'actually being out of that system and being on the side of advocacy is... liberating because you are not restricted'* (Bernard 2008, August 19; Olive 2007, November 7; Morgan 2015). She had opted out of a career structure and become an advocate to be more effective in the espousal of the rights of the other. Building on the principles there, I will now listen to voices in which I discern spiritual aspects to be more prominent in the creative conversation.

In keeping with the section title, I want to pursue the theme of independence and power, which I examined in 4.3.1., and illuminate points made about advocates versus the system by considering the nature of the influence they exercise. I wish to apply points theologically in response to Q3 (about what resources to *use* to answer questions), uncovering the virtuous and spiritual roots of independent advocacy, and ask how they can further assist the client and the advocate. Quotations from participants were classified under the 'live' category 'powerful,' firstly, based on two advocates (Janine and Nebi) who reflected their sense of powerlessness vis-à-vis medical professionals and the role that they played for their clients in their encounter with the system:

> *I think there is sometimes a belief that advocates hold some kind of power that realistically actually we don't... I guess, there is a sense in which we are very restricted realistically in what we can do, we don't hold any power at all... we don't have a clinical training...* (Janine 2007, October 1)

Janine's description of the power, or the lack of it, which she possessed was revealing of a view which an advocate took of herself. How can someone without power empower others? What is the nature of this self-effacing use of influence? In view of what has been said previously about advocacy skills and the developing profession of statutory advocacy services, it may be argued that Janine's view was rhetorical. That is, she did not want to represent herself as 'powerful' because the influence she would have as an advocate should have been properly instructed and should also be under the control of the partner or client. However, a non-instructed advocate defending the best interests of a client can have a considerable amount of leverage in the information which is given, always with consent, to a decision-maker about a partner's possible move or her serious medical treatment. Perhaps the clue to the power which advocates exercise was contained in Janine's expression *'restricted,'* which could also mean 'properly directed.' It was the focus of the limited action which she took, as an instructed advocate, which constituted the 'Reconstructed Empowerment' which she exercised. Nebi was adamant that it was not possible for clients to relate to ward staff as they do to advocates:

> N: *Yes, it's completely impossible… they cannot have the same sort of relationship… It's always the doctor on the ward who has the power to prescribe or discharge.* (Nebi 2007, October 22)

The above showed the actual relative vulnerability of advocates within the system, especially in relation to consultant psychiatrists in mental health, let alone how disadvantaged patients or clients may feel. But then, becoming representatively vulnerable for those vulnerable in real life may be an Action Based on Equality, according to the scheme I advance. This can be linked with what Bernard was told by an NHS manager—that chaplains were regarded as *'useless'* in the system. In spite of this, Bernard felt a transforming and transcending purpose in his advocating role (Bernard 2008, August 19). In many ways, this was similar for advocates although it can be observed that Nebi strongly represented their empowering function on the mental health ward. This evidence should be weighed alongside the fact that the IMCA and IMHA services, through their statutory place in decision-making for advocacy clients (from April 2007 and April 2009 respectively), did actually acquire new legal powers. The downside for informal mental health patients was that this development at that time could have meant less funding for non-instructed advocacy.

In answer to direct questions about motivations, firstly from an advocate, secondly from the member of a self-advocacy group, it was revealing to note the positive connotations in the use of 'power-based' words by workers to explain their feelings when advocating for clients or being supported in a position of powerlessness:

> *It's satisfaction when you get results and see someone quite happy. And, kind of, we don't have any power but we can empower them and I think, you know, that is why I continue doing my job.* (Jana 2007, October 22)

With Jana it was not possible to attribute a narrowly spiritual meaning to her words but '*satisfaction*' in results and seeing clients happy were an incentive with strong moral content. These were linked with the information-providing and signposting role which mental health advocates fulfil. The sense that Jana was drawn into the role of 'empowering' and changed by this can be described as RE. In the next example I look at the experience on the receiving end of advocacy, that of the self-advocate:

> (Co-f = Co-facilitator)
> *Co-f: How do you feel when you're in the group together? How does that make you feel?*
> *M: Good, good.*
> *P: Talk to people, talk to them, have a good experience, make a good idea so people with learning disability can say things, people need friends, people need colleagues, people like us, it's so good, I'm powerful... I'm taking over your job (Laughter...)* (Louise et al. 2007, November 23).

Here the speaker was acting as a spokesperson for four other self-advocacy group members. It demonstrated how the self-advocacy group provided the opportunity for one of its members to express publicly (to me as a researcher and a stranger) how empowered Pixy felt about the support she received from the group. The views of self-advocacy clients, (or 'advocacy partners') were important in assessing the practice. Enhancing the well-being of another through offering support is an activity which borders on the spiritual. A number of these examples can be linked to the Christian theme of 'looking to the interests of others.' St. Paul, when speaking of Jesus of Nazareth, wrote that, although he was 'in the form of God… emptied himself, taking the form of a slave' (Philippians 2:4–11, Bible). This overall theme of a Judaeo-Christian God subjecting himself to human needs, or the way an advocate can subject his ego to the demands of the service of another, was alluded to by another participant in relation to Buddhist thinking (Bull 2008). It is a tendency captured in the theme of RE. Taking from this the religious *motif* of emptying oneself for the benefit of the other, the diminished and submitted place of the ego can be connected with what I want to describe as 'Deep Advocacy.'[1]

A few of these examples, supplemented by that of the comparison between a chaplain's and an advocate's role, provided some evidence for a 'spiritual,' if not a theological, approach to advocacy, in which ego was subject to client needs. Putting the client or self-advocate at the centre of decisions is a process I described as 'Reconstructed Empowerment.' Jana's statement (above) that her motivation related to the *'satisfaction when you get results and see someone quite happy,'* followed by the problematic claim, *'we don't have any power but we can empower them,'* are relevant. While independent advocacy has progressed in occupying a clear space whereby decision-makers have legally to take account of statutory advocates and there is some kind of power (e.g. with the IMCA role), in many areas (generic mental health advocacy) the actual power which advocates had was related to the potential in the relationship between the client (or 'partner') and in the area they were being supported to negotiate. This included the validation of the advocacy function by professionals in the social work context. The way unpaid advocates used their space for their clients' advantage was striking when Norah and Bella talked about their independence of other services and the freedom that not being paid gave them; as Bella said, she would have to be honest and *'if the choice came*

---

[1] What I have defined as Reconstructed Empowerment is helpfully developed in a book section entitled, 'The Empty Self.' Drawing on the silence or lack of mental capacity in certain clients, Gammack (2011) wrote that 'deep advocacy' is 'empathic imaginative connectedness, where there is a reaching out beyond and below the prescriptions of the *status quo* to be in touch with the most profound longings of the silent ones… Deep advocacy is a practical theology of creativity… empathic indwelling, the faculty of sensing one's way into the self of the other' (Gammack 2011a, pp. 243–8). I find the expression 'empathic imaginative connectedness' apposite, and that it lines up with certain desirable conditions already evoked, such as being able to 'think around corners' (Kevin 3.2(a)).

between (a) party line and doing the best... for the person,' she would go for the person. As she said, she felt she would not lose her job, whatever she did (Norah and Bella 2009, December 14).

In citizen advocacy, where the advocate may be a volunteer, there was a strong link with the partner. This was divorced from the advocacy provider as some participants said they would put the relationship with the partner before loyalty to the organisation, as was the case with Bella (above). It was in these variations that the empowerment process was seen to be 'reconstructed,' constituting the description Reconstructed Empowerment. These constructive approaches to powerlessness, namely achieving results in self-advocacy or advocacy activity through the renunciation of patronising tactics in favour of clear arguments based on the needs of the other, could be allied more closely with collective ancient religious philosophies. The Judaeo-Christian model of responsibility and love towards one's neighbour can be as relevant to the practice as are relatively recent individual human rights-based approaches. This argument will be developed more fully later.

Moving on, in this second section I will consider perceptions of the relationships inherent in advocacy practice based on this independent empowered stance which has been outlined. But again they will come from the client perspective and be related back to the argument as they touch on Q3 and other SQs (Appendix 1). Once more in this section I will use lengthier quotations to highlight the views of clients in context, sometimes with more input from interviewers in order to elicit meaning and present fuller portraits of them. I facilitate analysis by drawing out the spiritual implications of these observations.

3   Deep Advocacy[2]: Connecting Clients, Self-Advocates and Advocates

Focusing on the rapport between different players, I follow again the professionalisation debate, this time from the client perspective via the context of a number of the SQs (1, 3 and 4). I discuss the role of self-

---

[2] I have borrowed the term both from George Gammack (Gammack 2011a, p. 240) and from the 'Deep Church' conversation begun by Professor Andrew Walker et al. The term Deep

advocates, the necessity and purpose of advocacy and how as a movement it faces social fragility. The qualities of listening and communication (from above) are particularly evident in the encounters I will analyse as well as the range of advocacy interventions which clients may experience. These are recounted by advocates at the end of the chapter. I will identify the 'caring gap' which independent advocacy addresses and how the voices of clients define a deeper advocacy experience and practice. Deep Advocacy, although it can be simple in its most basic form (see Sam, 4.1 (d) (iii)) above, was described above as 'empathic imaginative connectedness' (Gammack 2011a, pp. 243–8). I have defined empathy above as 'the ability to project oneself.' Returning for a moment to explain (from a distinctively Christian angle here) the value of the 'Deep Church' model, Walker (Walker 2003; Walker and Bretherton 2007) picked up Lewis' words and argued for a galvanisation of the 'Church' into action which overcomes its division along party lines:

> One of the distinguishing marks of Deep Church is that as adopted brothers and sisters of the incarnate Son of God what holds true for Him is intended to be normative for us... (Walker 2003, p. 20)

So in the developing conversation, I want to propose that the voices I attend to are together expressive of a spiritual, compassionate and self-sacrificial intention. This links with the advocacy movement's 'prefigurative' origins and can thus be heard as 'Deep Advocacy.'

How were clients referred to, or did they refer themselves to advocacy organisations, in particular in regard to the clients of Islingham Self-Advocacy Project (ISAP)? One of this number, Micky, said that he wanted to join the group (Micky et al. 2008, May 14). The co-interviewer, who also knew Micky, was thus able to translate his meanings, namely, that

---

Church was first coined by C.S. Lewis in a letter to the *Church Times* (Feb 8th 1952): he took a supernatural view of the message of Christianity which he then felt strongly was being undermined by liberal or 'modernist' streams in theology:

To a layman it seems obvious that what unites the Evangelical and the Anglo Catholic against the "Liberal" or "Modernist" is something very clear and momentous, namely, the fact that both are thoroughgoing supernaturalists, who believe in the Creation, the Fall, the Incarnation, the Resurrection, the Second Coming, and the ... Last Things. This unites them not only with one another but also with the Christian religion as understood *ubique et ab omnibus*. (C.S. Lewis 1952; Walker 2003, p. 20)

a personal connection with the advocacy support worker had motivated him to join. Yolanda was similarly drawn to the group. She started coming because she was told '*it was very interesting*' (Micky et al. 2008, May 14). Barry, however, appeared to count other more complex, even political, reasons for his involvement:

> *Barry: The reason is… because about two years ago the DDA, which is the Disability Discrimination Act. Anybody can go to the shop and they can't say you are too old or they don't like your race, that's discrimination. And then, after that, we done another one. I can't remember the other one we did*
> *Co-facilitator: Disability discrimination act… Equality duty and also… the Mental Capacity Act…* (Micky et al. 2008, May 14)

The factors which Barry mentioned, such as the Disability Discrimination Act (DDA) and the MCA, insofar as they affected clients, were elaborated upon in more detailed accounts, for example, Yolanda's narrative later in this chapter. From another organisation or data source, HEARTH, Whitney, a younger member who needed help with accommodation, was impressed by the volume of support which she was offered:

> *Whitney: It was quite interesting, every week, she's the one, she's helping… like, things like, writing things down, all the details, so each day, say Monday Tuesday Wednesday Thursday and Friday…*
> *Co-f: Did you get referred to advocacy by somebody? Who referred you?*
> *W: I think it was… was it Kieran*
> *Co-: Did your parents, was it your mum, say, who talked to an advocate or was it a carer, or care manager or social worker who talked to advocacy?*
> *W: I think it was my keyworker.* (Louise et al. 2007, November 23)

The relationship with the advocate, as she assisted Whitney with time management, seemed to be formed as part of the support process. Other referrals came from social workers and, for instance, in the case of Michael, finding a home was one of the crucial decisions which self-advocacy support workers (in these extracts) or advocates assisted with:

> *Michael: (speaks and signs using Makaton)*

Co-f: The care manager referred you... [short fault with recording equipment]

Co-f: What do you think is the most important things that an advocate needs to do?

Michael: (speaks)

Co-f: You find what they do is good... what's important about advocacy, what should an advocate do for you?

Michael: (speaks)

Co-f: (translating) Help you find a home

F: Thanks, Michael. (Louise et al. 2007, November 23)

This was also the case for Norma, a woman whose membership in ISAP helped her to develop her own support skills, who stated clearly her understanding of the role in terms of advocates being people who help you... *'to find places to live in... to help... get and find work...'* (Micky et al. 2008, May 14). And Whitney, again, identified the process by which an advocate signposted her to information and supported her to move:

W: They want to help... all of us here... and at [name of sub-project] things like Tim, I know Tim because he's my advocate and he starts helping me find some information about housing so I've got [name of sub-project], what they did, they moved me into [name of road] and they got my interview then; and after that I moved in January, I went to [name of road], they moved me in there. They interviewed me again, my meetings, and they are there for me, and then in the income support, what things like they do my housing, things like that. (Louise et al. 2007, November 23)

Finding a home, employment and income were therefore areas in which people connected with and appreciated the activity of advocates. Here it was important to recognise the continuum of advocacy (mentioned above by Kevin) as members of self-advocacy groups were also seen to be engaged in an advocacy role themselves. Robert and Yolanda emphasised the specific support that could be given to people as they required it in the course of their lives:

F: What do you see is important about being a self-advocate, or doing self-advocacy?

Barry: Having someone to speak up for you.

F: Right, thanks, Barry, what's the difference between advocacy and self-advocacy?

Barry: Advocacy is when you help people out... you help people, you know

F: anyone else want to say something about self-advocacy; any examples of how you have spoken up for yourself or the group and seen things change?

Yolanda: When we went to [name of hospital] once... they were talking about the changes they were going to do there... and how it affects them. (Micky et al. 2008, May 14)

Yolanda demonstrated the distinction between advocacy (as support received) and self-advocacy in supporting others with a greater level of disability than themselves, when she said '*they were talking about the changes... and how it affects them.*' Yolanda also showed awareness of the continuum and implied that she valued the interaction of their group with long-stay hospital patients. Others mentioned the difference between the two modes. The voices of participants and the co-facilitator distinguished between these in this more lengthy quotation. Whitney and Michael put it in this way:

Co-f: *altogether... so what you do with [name of project] is friends, and you work together as friends... but what's the difference between [name of project] together, and having an advocate like Nick and what you do with Nick, as your advocate?*

W: It's different, totally different... you want to talk to Nick on your own but you can't share it out with the meeting because it's your personal, personal business...

M: (speaks)

W: It's like me for instance, I know, I know Karen very well, I come here every day, Wednesdays and Fridays and I come to see Nick my advocate. He used to work in this borough in [name of charity] where people are learning things on their own in that independent way. They choose, they can choose their life, and they get their own flats, we get more confidence, and what I do, so for me for instance I looked at a place, then they turned it down for me, and this time, well they are going to set it out for me, so that's a one-bedroom flat, a studio...

Co-f: So Nick helps you with those things, and you that with Nick 'cause it's about your life, it's confidential isn't it? So is that different to what you do when you are at [name of project]?

W: It's what friends are for, have relationships together... talk about all our families and that, and where you are from

Co-f: Share things... (Louise et al. 2007, November 23)

It was evident that both Whitney and possibly Michael, related to Karen, the coordinator of the self-advocacy group and to Nick, an advocate, in different ways. This showed the subtle differences between roles in advocacy practice and the value of choices and relationships in the engagement of the practitioner. The progression from using the services of an advocate, to being a self-advocate, to a place where *'people are learning things on their own...'* was defined by Whitney. In terms of this engagement, it became apparent that it was not only the nature and depth of activity of the contact of the client with an advocate or an organisation but the period of time spent by the client in advocacy which influenced the quality of that relationship. For Louise the relationship with advocacy began when she was at school. She explained her involvement journey:

Louise: *Well, [name of project] take you to meetings, make sure you are in time for meetings, I've been into advocacy for a very long time, too long now, I did it from when I was at school and college, um, cos it wasn't based here it was based in [name of location]*

F: How did you get to hear about it at school?

L: Cos I was not that, I was not very happy at home so I talked to someone and since then I have been involved in advocacy

F: Was that someone an advocate themselves?

L: Yes. (Louise et al. 2007, November 23)

Other practitioners drew attention to this factor of the long-term link. I have already mentioned the solidity of the connection which advocates Norah and Bella saw as essential in their practice (see Sect. 6.1, below). This was further reflected upon by observations from Kevin in relation to his perception of advocacy practice as *'a constant revisiting'* as historically it moved on from *'focusing on citizen advocacy, which is closer to what I do for my neighbour.'* While this has been maintained, other services and statutory professional advocacy services were developed. Kevin pursued his point:

> *... at the same time I think we are beginning to revisit some of the really strong community focuses and some of the questions about how it is we build community for people... I boasted, 'We have these citizen advocates and the people they advocate for, they are the only ones who they have chosen to be with and they are not paid... our services are big and strong and essential...' Then I realised that this was an utter failure on our part, that we had advocated for some of those people for a long period of time and yet for some, their community connections, their kinship, their friendships were no stronger than when we started.* (Kevin 2008, January 14)

Kevin pinpointed the danger that professional advocacy would fail if it did not empower individuals to be responsible for their own friendships and held up the value of *'strong community focuses'* which resided to some extent in classic citizen advocacy, as we have already seen in relation to the doctrine of Wolfensberger. Further to this, Peter illustrated the prospect of failure in the area of learning disability when individuals left long-term hospital care because it was perceived as *'institutional'* but found that expected social support networks in the community were deficient because *'changes in learning disability services have no interest in people's social relationships as there was in the long stay hospital.'* Although he admitted there were a lot of things which were wrong in these hospitals which have now all been closed in England, there was nonetheless *'an emphasis on long-term relationships and culture and traditions, and all those things in which people had an expectation of what happens....'*

> *I suppose I'm seeing people go into services where that is being replaced by nothing, there's less people coming to the Christmas party, there are less people working on Christmas day. It's been that the brave new world of community care has not been working, we know it's not working...* (Peter 2008, December 9)

From the point of view of mental health, the chaplain Bernard underlined a point he made several times about the value of a settled community and the continuity that this represented compared with *'the new directives'* which involved moving into *'larger society.'* He considered that people were *'being encouraged to move out...'*

> *but that sometimes means that continuity (is lost)... I think that's one of the things we offer and people haven't got that in their lives at all. The rude word is dependency but it's really where are the reliable people and places I can come to when I need to, not all the time but when I need to, but that's been my model for our department but you wonder in future what's going to happen about that actually, and that perhaps more formal advocacy might miss out on that, you know getting to know people and being available, and I don't know how you do that really except for just being about the place...* (Bernard 2008, August 19)

In different ways and for different client groups, Peter and Bernard regretted the impact that government initiatives, such as personalisation, or the advantages of 'independent supported living' or 'care in the community' were having on individuals. Vulnerable people, especially those with learning disabilities, moving into the community, they seemed to imply, meant that absorption in localities was not easily facilitated. Importantly, Bernard pinpointed the deficit and fragmentation in social and spiritual support which formal professionalised advocacy may not currently address for mental health clients: *'getting to know people and being available.'* And Kevin had stated earlier that advocacy did not always get it right in countering these trends, or in working with individuals to ensure that their status in a new community was enhanced or so that they were sufficiently empowered. I have illustrated some of the definitions from Chaps. 2 and 3 by showing the range of advocacy interventions which clients experience and the depth at which advocates are expected to work; I have also covered the 'mixed mode' by which some individuals with advocates may be self-advocates (form part of support groups), or may indeed be peer advocates themselves, on an unpaid or possibly paid basis. In this section I have shown how the basics of advocacy can assist vulnerable individuals to live peaceably in community. I will develop this point specifically about 'Deep Advocacy' in community, which is a response to **SQ3**, more sharply in Sects. 3.3 and

3.4 of Chap. 6. But in the next section I suggest from the service-user perspective how self-advocacy can make a deep and lasting difference in lives, through RE.

4   Self-Advocates Take Control and Share Views on Social Life and Representation

I said, "This has got to stop, you can't keep doing things like this to women" (Yolanda)

I will begin by placing the first example from the participant in its social context. For the ISAP focus group interview, of which Yolanda was part, I built on the experience with HEARTH. With the former I discussed issues such as mental capacity in greater detail. Here I will concentrate on examples of how the group were empowered in their self-advocacy and then look at an extended example from Yolanda's experience as a narrated case within this section. Firstly, with the aid of the tutor, the co-facilitator, the group discussed a DVD they had watched about an individual moving house with the support of an advocate:

> *Barry: They wanted to shift her out of her own home and put her in a care home but she did not like it… so they got social services and an advocate called Jenny…*
> *Co-f: Did Laura have capacity?*
> *Barry: I should think she did… but she couldn't speak, she did it by non-verbal, signs…*
> *…*
> *Yolanda: We enjoyed watching it because we felt really sorry for her; being shifted from her own home and then to be moved to a place where she sat watching a television, where a rude lady came in and switched it over. She just switched it over without telling any of them and none of them could speak up and say to her: 'I was watching that.' (Micky et al. 2008, May 14)*

ISAP acted like a trade union for members of the learning community representing their concerns to the college board, and it was therefore interesting to note both the curriculum they were exposed to and the views and opinions engendered. This particular example linked with the discussion above about challenging stigma in relation to people with learning disabilities. There were also parallels with the data from HEARTH (and Pixy's account) in relation to the view of the character of advocates. Einstein noted, as we saw above, that when *'somebody helps you it makes you feel good,'* and Madonna that *'It feels good to help each other, anybody can help each other'* (Micky et al. 2008, May 14). Einstein also advised that you have *'got to have the right people'* to perform this role and that it is *'about people making their own choices'* (Micky et al. 2008, May 14). Although not possible here, this insight relates to the understanding of self-directed support (SDS) (Hampshire-County-Council 2008) whereby service-users choose their own staff to employ.

This extended example, a testimony from Yolanda, demonstrated the effect of the self-advocacy group in terms of social confidence and the ability to take control in an allegation she had made about a colleague:

> *There was a man at work who kept harassing me and I came home and I told my carer about it, and she said 'You have a word with Mr. [name] at work.' He kept doing it every day, and I told [name] when I got home and she said, 'You have another word with Mr. [name] and tell him and perhaps he will put [name] in his place,' so I did. Then he came in and said, 'Why did you tell Mr. [name] about me?' 'Look, [name] I said, this has got to stop, you can't keep doing things like this to women. And I said if it doesn't stop, my carer will be the next one talking to him. And do you know, what he then said wasn't very nice. He said, 'You do, and I'll hit you.' I said, 'Oh yes, you lay a hand on me, and I'll have the police on you.'*
> *Scoby: Well done*
> *Yolanda: And I said, 'I really mean it too, [name].' And he took one look at me, and guess what, he never did it again.* (Micky et al. 2008, May 14)

This powerful description of a clear action in a situation, which, if the individual had less capacity or, in this case less confidence to question the behaviours and consequently to champion allegations, could have led to a safeguarding (vulnerable) adult alert. Advocates may then have been involved, too. It shows successful use of a self-advocacy programme and illustrates how the campaigning social movement side of self-advocacy prevented the need to use social services (see SQ4). Of course, it is difficult to judge whether Yolanda's self-assertive approach was due to her personality and that this was why she belonged to ISAP, or whether it was her membership in the group which empowered her to stand up for herself as she did. What can be said is that the environment in which she felt comfortable enabled her to respond in this way and to describe publicly what she did. It is an example which reinforced the concept of RE of which I have already raised a number of instances.

Advocacy is about both empowerment and managing complaints successfully, so in fairness I need to be aware of critiques of advocacy. Often defects in one profession can be seen more clearly through the lens of a comparable profession. Below, I consider Qs 1 and 2, or how advocacy practice can be addressed within the framework of another similarly independent profession, that of chaplaincy. Chaplains or spiritual care coordinators are distinguished by their independence from services in a different way from advocates, but have similarities in terms of their frequency of deployment in health and social care. Their voices suggest that their role encompasses advocacy although for spiritual and religious care they occupy a more specific dimension. On the way to that place I want to listen to voices from chaplaincy and advocacy as they critique each other, but I begin with a quasi-statistical comparison of their known recent deployment in England.

5   Spiritual Critiques of Advocacy Practice

5.1   The Possible Overlapping Roles of Advocates and Chaplains

I want to suggest an integrated model of advocacy practice based on spiritual and cultural elements by making comparisons and correlations (in addition to those already made between advocates vis-à-vis self-advocates and clients). Although this book in principle relates to qualitative research, contrasts between spiritual care coordinators or chaplains and advocates may at this stage be enhanced by some relevant figures. For numbers of full-time equivalent (FTE) chaplains, figures showed that at the beginning of 2010 there were around 425 full-time and approximately 3000 part-time chaplains employed by the National Health Service. In addition there were 'numerous volunteer chaplains of all denominations and faiths' (Hospital-Chaplaincies-Council 2010, p. 5).[3] Against this, it was more difficult to discover numbers of FTE advocates because it was not yet known exactly how many services there were nationally. This, according to Martin Coyle, then Head of Quality and Development at A4A, was because there was 'no obligation for groups to record or report this data,' which would include the number of volunteer and of part-time advocates. Also, there were a number of organisations who said their work included advocacy where the services listed did not appear to reflect this appropriately and, vice versa, a few who may be providing advocacy without describing it as such. However, on the basis that every local authority in England (and Wales) must provide the statutory services of IMCAs and IMHAs and an aggregation of numbers of advocates depending on known provider organisations, the following figures emerged.

With approximately 600–800 advocacy organisations in the country, an educated estimate would suggest an average of eight advocates per group, and this would indicate a total number in the range of 4800–6400. It was also unclear what effect the variable of volunteer advocates would have on this number, in the same way as it was for chaplains. There was not a definitive list of trained IMHAs or IMCAs—which must be provided in every local authority—but estimates of the number of trained IMCAs tended to be around 500. It would be reasonable to assume a similar number for IMHAs, according to Coyle (2010) although commissioning patterns across the country made this assumption unclear (Coyle 2010; see Morgan 2011b).

During discussion of a case study at a conference, in which the example of a young man with learning disabilities undergoing treatment in 2007 was described, Oliver, a chaplain, reflected that the IMCA service had not yet been introduced at the time of the critical incident and that he had

---

[3] Compare this with statistics gathered by chaplain Imam Siddiq Diwan of 391.2 FTE, possibly representing a decline (Diwan 2015).

supported healthcare professionals in a decision to treat the patient when the family were displaced. He noted that an IMCA was now needed, so that a chaplain was superfluous or could not be used because they were employed by the trust. Contrasting with the perceptions of chaplains Dorothy and Nigel above, Oliver felt that it was a shame that many of the roles of the chaplain had been eroded away by the PALS office in his trust and advocacy. *'I'd love to be an IMCA,'* he stated, *'and I have a gut feeling that advocates have taken over traditional areas of involvement for chaplains'* (T. Oliver 2012).

Given the background of a possible increase in advocacy provision compared with chaplains/spiritual care coordinators, there were signs that both disciplines may have practices and training which they could beneficially share. The above proposal of twin best practices principles, Action Based on Equality and RE can assist with such a project and encourage the vulnerable to be safer in the community. When a vulnerable individual is at risk and more unfortunate consequences ensue, the health and social care systems are interrogated and advocacy may well be involved. In the next section of this chapter, I will consider some challenges to advocacy practice. As an emerging profession, advocacy schemes contract with their clients and have complaints procedures which they set out when they are working in a non-instructed way.

5.2   Chaplains Evaluate Advocacy: Complaints, the Smoking Ban and 'Face Value'

The staff say, "The patients have more rights than we do" (Dorothy); I don't think it's enough to take the patient's side (Colin)

The empowering and rights-based functions of advocacy were underlined by some of the understandings of spiritual care coordinators, but they were also questioned, as I will show in examples below. I seek a deeper approach to independent advocacy incorporating Reconstructed Empowerment and Action Based on Equality. For instance, the chaplain Nigel stated he was aware of such services and said that if he knew *'formal advocacy services'* existed, he would in fact use them *'in the first instance.'*

But where no such service exists, then I feel it is part of my role to take that up and to do it as best I can. But I wouldn't be following any formal advocacy protocols in doing so. I'd be doing it in my intuitive sort of way... (Nigel and Colin 2008, September 11)

The primacy which Nigel and Colin gave to advocates was reflected elsewhere by Sarah, who surprised me when she said she felt that advocates worked *'quite separately from us, because they are kind of more active'*:

They are... are, I want to say, front-line, you know and I like to think we work more behind the scenes, really that's my experience, I know that's not the case for all chaplains but they (advocates) have more of a voice, I think
F: Really?
S: I think so, yeah, I mean it's not to say I wouldn't have a voice if I wanted to have one if I felt it was necessary but I think they are more speaking to the patient... (Sarah and Karim 2008, December 4)

This interesting observation from Sarah, that advocates appeared to her to be on the 'front-line' and to have a voice, was based on good knowledge. In mental health advocacy, as we shall see further below, the issue of voice and the empowerment (RE) which was drawn from the social situation of advocates was crucial. Karim's view also linked his awareness of the existence of advocates with his own approach to the support of patients:

K: I sometimes see patients who appeal to advocates to help them express their views; we know the same patients but I think we are dealing with a different aspect... (Sarah and Karim 2008, December 4).

Turning to more critical and analytical perspectives in accordance with Q2, Dorothy was a spiritual care coordinator and manager of nearly 20 years' experience. Her experience of advocates was not extensive, but her initial view of advocates was that their main role was to make complaints. I believe her view changed in the course of our conversation.

Material from the interview provided two narrated examples which I will analyse. The first one concerned a patient with a complaint which the advocate mentioned to the ward round and which he was told to deal with himself. Dorothy took up the story, describing how a female patient had gone into the ward round to complain about the chaplain *'and was told that she needed to deal with it herself.'* Dorothy commented, *'How awful that she was told she had to do that herself!'*

> *So she ended up with the advocate who sent the letter out… perfectly fine, as it turned out… I felt though that there were two things that needed to be held in tension, one was to do with the particular person, who we knew well, we knew her and her material, and we knew that she was likely to attribute more… than was actually in it…* (Dorothy 2008, September 18)

Dorothy was concerned that the patient's voice had not been heard since the *'chaplain needed to recognise that he had gone over a boundary with this particular patient'* so she was *'left feeling at the end of this particular complaint'* that it was due to the patient's voice having *'been taken away.'*

> *'What I was concerned to do in addressing the complaint was to give her, her voice back.'*

I then clarified that there was also an issue about a patient not being heard at that ward round and that Dorothy thought it should have been dealt with then since she was *'left feeling if the ward round had said they wanted to speak to me as the manager, the complaint could have been dealt with in a better way, as more helpful to the patient.'* (Dorothy 2008, September 18)

The complaints process was used rather than going straight to the manager of that service, namely Dorothy. In raising the complaint, the patient was supported by the advocate. This reflection on the process of advocacy seemed more critical of the ward round than the practice of the advocate. Dorothy felt that the complainant's *'voice had been taken away'* and she was concerned to give her that *'voice back.'* In fact, she seemed to be suggesting that she felt that she had been prevented from being an advocate for the patient by the action of the ward and the advocate. However, although I could not speak to the ward round or the advocate, it could also be argued that the advocate was carrying out a clear supportive role as an independent person, supporting the writing of a letter in relation to the ward round's issue with the chaplaincy. This is evidence of an ambiguity in the role of the advocate (in answer to SQ5) because Dorothy was not able to be an independent advocate as she also spiritually supported the staff as an NHS employee. Dorothy had other concerns with advocacy practice, as she saw it. When Dorothy was asked about the nature of the profession, she indicated that she was concerned about the assertion of rights by advocates:

> D: *Now I see that advocacy is a movement and it needs to be a profession. The reason I say I think it is a movement is that advocacy has about it an element of campaigning for user rights, and therefore the advocate is talking to the user in an attempt to assert rights, um…*

She was worried that this was as *'exploitative of the user as, or risks being as exploiting of the user as whoever is deemed to be not treating them very well.'* This was why Dorothy summarised that advocacy had a *'campaigning edge'* (Dorothy 2008, September 18). Dorothy explained her concern in more detail and related the explanation to the incident above and the way in which advocacy can cause patients to be handled differently:

> D: *The advocate has put in a lot of complaints and… you know the nurses can't help themselves but feel we better handle this patient with kid gloves otherwise they will put in a complaint, and therefore the patient gets handled defensively with the best will in the world. They may not be uncaring, it may just be, we're going to abide by the rules in relation to this patient because otherwise the advocate will be on our back.*
> F: *So they might be behaving in a less human, less responsive way, reflecting on it…*
> D: *It makes them too self-conscious*
> F: *Yea, that's really interesting…*
> D: *Which is why I think it should be a profession because if it's a well-established discipline, then I think that need to campaign will not be there* (Dorothy 2008, September 18)

The emphasis on the rights of the patient, rather than responsibility for the well-being of the staff, meant that the role of the advocate was skewing the treatment of a patient on the ward and making staff behave in a *'less human… way.'* This could be a shortcoming if a patient with an advocate was treated more harshly, but the *'defensive'* treatment Dorothy mentioned needed exploring. The advocacy role was apparently distinctive from that of the chaplain, the former characterised by a more independent and individual-centred approach, which was often human rights-based. By contrast, chaplains looked to serve the whole of the community, staff included. Dorothy's criticism of advocacy practice was in this sense understandable. Turning again to rights, smoking on mental health wards is now only possible outside on NHS premises, and again for Dorothy the question of rights was prominent in the second critical incident she outlined:

> D: ... it's a human right to smoke, however in a mental health situation where people have been sectioned, they have been detained against their will, usually for their protection so they have a human right to smoke, a human right also not to get cancer, but, um, it leaves us with a dilemma, and it's a very complicated issue and I think I have been party to a lot of discussions where the trump card is expected to be that it's a human right to smoke, and I feel that it cannot be... (Dorothy 2008, September 18)

She explained further that there was not anywhere for patients to smoke so they have to be taken downstairs specially. Furthermore, Dorothy related, a member of staff was seriously hurt when escorting a patient downstairs. With some anger, she asserted that it was a human right to smoke no less than it was a human right not to be killed at work. The question was how to balance those rights (Dorothy 2008, September 18). Patients—and possibly advocates on their behalf, although she did not say so—who were on the second floor of the building had demanded the right to be escorted downstairs in order to smoke. On account of the injury there was understandably reluctance on the part of the staff to do this. Dorothy identified this as a clash: *'it's a human right to smoke, and it's a human right not to be killed at work,'* and pleaded for advocates to be more sophisticated and to take a holistic approach (Dorothy 2008, September 18). Dorothy's view of advocacy was summed up as *'not necessarily... very helpful'* because complaints were lodged after an advocate's visit to a ward without any *'kind of sifting':*

What she's done is, she's arrived and spoken to someone who is really very unwell and has taken at <u>face value</u> all the complaints that the patient has made. The problem is that particular ward is politically sensitive for a whole range of reasons, and therefore the complaint takes on a greater significance than it really has, and it contributes to… to lowering staff morale to a very large extent, to the extent that the staff say the patients have far more rights than we do. And whether that's perception or not, I can see how they arrive at that perception, and that's very largely due to the advocate. That's not the only factor. But that's quite a factor in it. (Dorothy 2008, September 18)

The criticism of the advocate's practice was highly ambivalent. A chaplain is an employee of the NHS trust which is also her paymaster, and she cares spiritually for staff as well as patients, as we saw above. The position is complex. As I have previously suggested, chaplaincy is a shade more 'independent'; later I suggest a median position (see (c) below). An independent advocate, however, seeks to represent and support a client and should use some judgement, but the role of a mental health advocate (if not an IMCA) is principally to be on the side of the client. In fact, Nebi underlined this by using the term 'face value' approvingly:

It's someone who takes what the service user says at <u>face value</u> and supports them. It doesn't matter that you condone… whatever fantasies they may have. You are a partner, an equal relationship, not a professional with, say, a duty of care of which you could subsequently be accused… (Nebi 2007, October 22)

In the interview I challenged Nebi's point since it seemed that there was a question whether the advocate was abdicating responsibility:

F: Not with a duty of care?
    N: Yes, but I am saying it would be good to have a duty of care which isn't like what a social worker has, you are already in a very good position not to give advice, not to act in the best interests approach so at the end of the day you are doing different work so if someone is asking for discharge, you support them not because you know they are not well enough to be turned out but because they want it and you leave the judgement of whether they are well enough to professional doctors… (Nebi 2007, October 22)

In this section I have focused on the views of non-advocates on advocacy practice, but I also analysed their views alongside the views of advocates and used my own experience to place them into context with examples. In respect of Dorothy's account, more information would be required in order to say whether the advocate had done a good job, but it would not be appropriate for an independent advocate (as opposed to a chaplain) to attend to staff morale. There was no particular evidence that the advocate was doing a poor job and later in the interview Dorothy herself pinpointed the need for the medium of advocacy since she was *'really unclear that reasonable judgements are being made about patients'* (Dorothy 2008, September 18).

5.3   Chaplaincy as a Provider of Advocacy

This section will provide a response to SQs 1 and 5 as I will consider the advocating role of chaplains and also look at the part which volunteers play. Turning to other spiritual care coordinators, Nigel commented on the role of the advocate as one he associated with raising complaints on the part of patients. However, unlike for Dorothy, his principle point was that the advocacy service has been taking on a role which chaplaincy previously performed:

> Nigel: *Well, I remember when I first came to [name of hospital], um, the chaplains were really the only group of people who held agenda-less reflection-groups for service-users who would be involved with elements of advocacy, kind of, just as a normal sort of part what might have been required, and particularly relationships, but with the development of the more, and I would include advocacy as a step in a parallel development, um, it's felt to me as a chaplain that some of the informal elements of my role, which I have really taken up because there was no-one else to do them, have now become located more objectively in other groups of people.* (Nigel and Colin 2008, September 11)

The *'agenda-less reflection groups for service users,'* was a development for which Nigel was grateful since the responsibility for this was now shared. The *'more active self-organising user culture'* Nigel mentioned was a feature highlighted above as important in its impact on advocacy. Colin spoke of referrals he had made to BAME-specific advocacy services, an aspect I also covered above:

> C: *When I work with someone who has a lot of agitation or a difficulty in accepting what has happened to them, and particularly again in one of our hospitals [name of hospital] where I have often referred people to [name of organisation], which is a black advocacy organisation, um, and encouraged them sometimes to get in touch with their parents sometimes, to get in touch with [name of organisation] for that sort of support, and to help them... otherwise I...*
>
> F: *How has that worked, the referrals to [name of organisation]?*
>
> C: *Well, [name of organisation] seem to be a fairly efficient organisation, by and large, and quite well-funded ... I know the people... I work in [name of town] anyway, who run it, and it's quite an impressive organisation.* (Nigel and Colin 2008, September 11)

Colin remarked on a particular advocacy service's efficiency, user focus and stable funding. He described an advocacy role he took on himself and the sort of activity an advocate will routinely carry out (whether instructed by a social worker or not) in contacting family. It should be noted, as stated above, that since this interview, the IMHA service now means a patient under a Mental Health section has that statutory right (from April 2009), a role which there is pressure to extend. Colin commented further on the recruitment policy of another service, quoted at some length because it illustrated the relationship between a chaplain and an advocate:

> *There's also I say I know there's one or two people I know, ex-users of the service, who are now advocates in [name of hospital], and so I would say [name] comes round, she's around Thursdays and Fridays if you want to have a word with her, but she normally goes to every patient and actually opens up the conversation...*
>
> F: *She's a volunteer?*
>
> C: *She's a volunteer... and opens up if there are any problems, and she tells them what their rights are, and she's quite forceful in doing (so) and 'You don't have to do this... you don't have to' and 'You just let me know.' And occasionally I find myself doing that also as well, you know, when people tell me which sec-*

tion they are on, whether it's Section 2 or Section 3, and I might just, you know... my knowledge is kind of limited... I am often asked you know to go in when the solicitor is there and things, to speak on their behalf. Again, that has to be balanced because mostly the users we are dealing with are in acute psychosis so therefore their expectations of you as a chaplain are that you have some kind of magic wand that will open the door for them and find a way out. (Nigel and Colin 2008, September 11)

The expectation that Colin should attend meetings is definitely the role of a mental health advocate. In view of the previous discussion about volunteer and citizen advocates, it was illuminating to see evidence of an apparently effective volunteer. Previously I noted that an advocate, Peter, was unconvinced about the value of training advocates as volunteers. In this case it appeared from Colin's words that she was modelling advocacy practice for him: *'She's quite forceful in doing (so) and "You don't have to do this... you don't have to" and "You just let me know."* And occasionally I find myself doing that also as well.'

A comparative analysis between the work of the chaplain and the advocate was the background to the interview and I noted similarities with terms which advocates used to describe their work: Nigel spoke of *'levelling out the imbalances of power,'* which I have previously synthesised with the terms which Janine and Sam used, namely, *'mouthpiece'* and *'equaliser.'*

Having approved of the fact that mental health advocates can be former service-users, the assessments Nigel, Colin and Dorothy made of the advocacy practice they were aware of are summed up in two direct quotations from them:

Nigel: 'I would say that the work of advocacy needs to be carried out by someone who is skilled and who has enough internal capacity to allow their experience to motivate them not get their experience mixed up....'

Colin: 'The advocate themselves ended up opposing the professionals in a way which I did not think really served them, or was to the benefit of the client... where it might need improvement are around this business of skill... I don't think it's enough to just take the patient's side...' (Nigel and Colin 2008, September 11)

Dorothy and Nigel and Colin all had similar objections to some of the behaviours of mental health advocates. The need to take the 'patient's side' was both a strength and a weakness, but it should be noted that the IMCA service was more subtle in the description of the 'best interests' process. The difference between medical best interests and person-centred best interests is often signalled by advocates, from my experience. However, for someone without capacity (which may be for someone under a Mental Health section as well) the best interests of a person may not be something for which the individuals themselves wish and may also be distinct from medical best interests. Zablon, a spiritual care coordinator whose voice we have already heard in relation to the discussion on advocacy and barriers of culture (2.3.2.) emphasised the need for good advocacy practice:

> *My experience as a chaplain and as a minister talking with patients really about their difficulties at a particular time, is that they... find that the doctors and other people do not really engage and listen, and they feel supported when there is someone, an independent person*
> *F: Can you just say, to clarify, whether you think they could be used more in the NHS than they are at the moment?*
> *Z: Yes, I think I would say that emphatically, I think, and also basically their role in another way is to allow the clinicians and the nurses to really understand what is going on, and so it's a two-way thing, and supporting the patients and making sure the patients understand the staff, and what is going on...* (Zablon 2008, September 19)

Not only did Zablon put forward the need for advocates to be engaged in an independent mediatory role but he saw the need for advocates to learn from the sort of advocacy interventions which chaplains engage in. When I asked him about what chaplains could do in terms of training advocates, he replied:

> *Z: We ought to have a slot, I think, to talk about what the chaplain does, what our understanding of mental health is, would be quite important, I think, for the team.*
> *F: Yes, that could work as well but there are people who are advocates who are not necessarily religiously motivated, they are often human-rights based...*

> *Z: Yes, the issue of religion, which is an asset for spirituality; we talk about religion as an aspect of spirituality; from our perspective even an agnostic has spirituality from meaning in life to hope in life so we can't leave it to religion as it were...* (Zablon 2008, September 19)

Zablon made the point that 'spirituality' rather than religion is a more unifying place for the discussion of theology and that deliberation on how people's spiritual needs cannot be fully met by organised religions as they are popularly conceived. The literature on this subject attests to Zablon's point (Flanagan and Davie 1995; Heelas and Woodhead 2007). But the purpose of this book is to go beyond these statements of orthodoxy from sociologists of contemporary religion in order to explore a robust and coherent Practical Theology for advocacy from within a spiritual tradition. This is the challenge which the evidence has raised and for which I will use philosophical as well as theological resources to try and meet.

It may be that it is precisely in books and articles linking spirituality and mental health, which I have previously outlined, that signposts may be found for the development of a more spiritually attuned approach to advocacy. Chaplains or spiritual care coordinators are distinguished by their independence from services in a different way from advocates and would certainly see their role as encompassing advocacy although spiritual and religious care has a more specific dimension. It may be good to consider a model for shared training or ways in which advocacy and chaplaincy practice can be usefully merged for learning. Such a project may benefit from a 'use of self' model which was developed in the chaplaincy service. This will show the interplay between advocacy and spirituality in a Practical Theological domain which could improve practice in both disparate disciplines.

5.4   Strengthening the Skills of Advocates Through the 'Use of Self'

In direct response to the Q3 regarding philosophical and theological models to understand advocacy and in continuation of the theme of putative training for advocacy practitioners, I will now adapt one reflective stance and refer back to the aspects of my method. The participant and chaplain Nigel set out an open approach and the possibility of combining advocacy and pastoral care training:

> *F: Are you aware of advocates having any particular training... Have you been involved... would you be open to that?... Because in IMCA we need to establish whether people have their views, preferences, beliefs and values represented...*
>
> *N: Yeah, it would fit very neatly into some of the training we already do, I mean we have an approach to training which I would describe as developing the use of self, and it would apply very nicely... to advocates... you want them to become more skilled in the use of themselves.* (Nigel and Colin 2008, September 11)

My questioning technique could have appeared to be 'leading.' I stated above that I was a practitioner as well as a researcher, that is a practising advocate and experienced minister of religion, and that part of my methodology was reflexive (as I have stated) so that there was no need to conceal that one issue I wished to consider was how chaplaincy and advocacy training could enrich each other. Being situated personally within the concerns of my research was an advantage, since I used my insider status to consider ways in which advocacy practice could be enhanced from a pragmatic point of view. This did not conflict with academic credibility and validity but belonged within it, and in fact illustrated the use of self.

The 'use of self' as a concept grew out of a theory from social psychology which came to be known as symbolic inter-actionism, whereby the self was defined in its re-action to others. It had many adherents including Mead, Peirce, Cooley and Goffmann. Arnd-Caddigan and Pozzuto (2008) stated that this had an influence on the psychologist and therapist, Carl Rogers (Arnd-Caddigan and Pozzuto 2008, p. 236).

Mackey described the 'sense of self' as growing out of bio-psycho-social being, which may include empirical data from neurobiology and therefore lead to improved practice. He continued, helpfully in this context, to identify a spiritual element in stating that our 'cognitive and emotional conception of who we are, is a spiritual phenomena (sic), invisible yet recognizable by us and by others. The word "spiritual" does not refer to a particular religious orientation but to a perspective on life that suggests a need within all human beings to find meaning in their lives that transcends observable realities' (Mackey 2008, pp. 226–7). Arnd-Caddigan and Pozzuto (2008) made points about contemporary community and how its impermanence, 'as noted by Taylor (1989), Sennett (1998) and Giddens (1991) has changed both the nature and awareness of self.' And for Mackey, the sense of self had been eroded by the change and variability to which post-modern life was subject (Mackey 2008, pp. 236–7).

Turning back to my material, as a background to his advancement of the 'use of self' in training, Nigel identified a problem in practice that *advocacy organizations may have a very simplistic view about how one uses one's own experience* in this unstable scenario (Nigel and Colin 2008, September 11).

> *The work of advocacy needs to be carried out by someone who is skilled and has enough internal capacity to allow their experience to motivate them but to not get their experience mixed up, or to allow their experience to be triggered... that requires specific formation for advocates who have been users of the service.*
> (Nigel and Colin 2008, September 11)

Interestingly in relation to Nigel's spiritual status, the case study Mackey used was pertinent to the same theme and involved a therapist using herself, a non-religious antagonist to patriarchal religion, to understand a client with a spiritual perspective:

> The therapist attempted and failed many times before she was able to resonate with Barbara's experiences, but once the resonance was reached Barbara was able to describe her world in a way that changed her experiences of her religion.
>
> This process of attempting, failing and attempting again on the part of the therapist is use of self... This change was not a mere change in attitude toward the religion to accommodate the client, but a feeling with the client that altered the clinician's understanding of herself, as she came to know Barbara's world. (Mackey 2008, pp. 240–241)

Returning to the chaplain Nigel, he observed that an approach to training which developed the 'use of self' could be very helpful to advocates so that they could be more *'skilled in the use of themselves.'* Although, as previously stated, advocacy is not the same as counselling or therapy, it could be beneficial on the above evidence to incorporate principles from counselling training such as working from *'the agenda of the other'* or *'the use of self'* into advocacy training. Nigel summarised the practice of chaplains in using their theological acumen to tackle spiritual issues with the use of self and surmised that it may assist advocacy practice.

> *We tend… to operate at a more technically esoteric level where direct spiritual, directly apprehended spiritual experience is common right across all religious cultures, so our own reflective practice is deepening our own exposure and understanding around that, and again it is summed up by the use of self. And I would have thought that sort of approach would be very useful in advocacy training.* (Nigel and Colin 2008, September 11)

Nigel's insight deserves further research outside the scope of this book. Further connection could be usefully made with theories clustered in areas of 'emotional labour,' compassionate care and resilience in nursing, and from similar reflection within chaplaincy (Hunter and Deery 2009; Kelly 2013; P. Smith 1992). In relation to the overall book, this 'use of self' may provide a guide for theological and spiritual discourse in an understanding of the functions of independent advocacy, as I have previously briefly summarised them as Reconstructed Empowerment and Action Based on Equality.

With an emerging spiritual or theological perspective (from 'outside'), which grew out of the dialogue with chaplains (as advocacy practitioners), and from other facets including advocates and clients which have previously been highlighted, I am in a position to move into the final section. After critiques levelled at advocacy by chaplains, one aspect from psychology ('use of self') was raised by a chaplain as a constructive resource, and so I will blend this with a return to some case examples of best practice which I have noted. The 'use of self' is implicit at this point as I consider approaches which advocates actually have taken in cultural and spiritual domains. I will therefore ponder more directly the perceptions on advocacy practice from those using advocacy skills and in relation to social, cultural and spiritual areas, and I will apply senses of Reconstructed Empowerment and Action Based on Equality, if appropriate, to ground the theme of Q3 and to show how it is possible to apply the principles at this stage and in retrospect to my account of the nature of the occupation. In this next section, voices of participants are thus allowed to speak on the topic of advocacy, patient and public involvement and personal, theological and spiritual development.

6   How Advocates Address Social, Cultural and Spiritual Support Needs

'Take someone's wishes... and find a practical solution' (Sam)

In the last part of the chapter I focus on the voices of participants, mostly advocates or spiritual care coordinators, whose contributions I grouped particularly according to social, cultural and spiritual domains. I will look at parallels between the work of advocates and chaplains/spiritual care coordinators and draw lessons for advocacy best practice and professional development in order to address Qs 2 and 3 according to the developing argument.

The reason for interviewing spiritual care coordinators or chaplains as well as advocates and their clients was to gain an insight into a professional view from a different angle. Of course, I could have chosen another healthcare profession, such as nurses or social workers or dramatherapists to engage with. All these would be principally employed by the NHS or local authorities and would not have been independent. It is true that chaplains are paid by the NHS, but they are also partially recruited and employed by the religious community which they represent: for example, an Anglican priest must hold a licence of the diocesan bishop to be selected, which explains the element of independence alluded to above.

As a spiritual care coordinator/chaplain working in a mental health trust, Bernard's general view of advocacy was that it was something which was needed although he did not immediately associate it with independence. In fact he identified a complaints service (PALS) funded by the trust as a provider of this, but this service could not by definition be independent. Earlier I considered the role of PALS within NHS trusts and considered that advocacy was needed above and beyond PALS, according to the SQ5. Bernard himself explained how he would, similarly to the chaplains above, after signposting advocacy services, if necessary, go to meetings to speak for patients. Bernard described his experience when I asked him what he thought advocacy consisted of:

> *Bernard: Well, I suppose my experience has been that it is often needed, and the need to encourage people to get advocacy for themselves, and to suggest ways through… Yes, and sometimes I personally will act as an advocate on behalf of a patient, or they want me to go to a meeting with them, speak for them because they don't feel confident to be able to do that for themselves… so in various ways I act as an advocate or refer people to people that can be…*
>
> *B: Well, I suppose that you are accessible to people and you give them space and confidence to speak about the problem as fully as they can because often they don't feel that they can do that. Um, and then to think about, um, supporting them, often saying, 'Do you think you can do this by yourself, or do you need support?' Because sometimes people, having spoken about it will say, 'I think I can further that myself.'* (Bernard 2008, August 19)

Bernard had positioned himself in terms of his spiritual vocation ('in' the system but not 'of' it), but, in relation to the negotiation of the precise pastoral, advocating role, Bernard focused on the fact that when he had discussed something through with an individual in his Trust, he found that they were able to advocate for themselves, or that he would just be in the meeting to 'underline things' (Bernard 2008, August 19). One activity which both chaplains and advocates carried out was letter-writing. Mental health advocates would often be asked by their clients to write letters to certain bodies (e.g. housing); Bernard referred to the fact that he may have needed to write letters for people when they could not attend meetings and to request explanations. This related to material above in addressing the stigmatising and powerless position acute psychiatric patients may find themselves in (see Chap. 2.3.1.-3.). Bernard noted that when he was working with individuals he was sometimes the person who had *'known them longer than many people in the (treatment) team'* (Bernard 2008, August 19).

6.1   Attachment, Spirituality and Community Stability

Professional advocates working with people with learning disabilities have also often been the only point of fixity for individuals when many social workers have come and gone. Norah noted above her attachment to someone she had supported for nearly 30 years:

> *I got very attached to the man I advocate for, I couldn't be without him, I think the balance has tipped a bit the way that he could manage without me quite well now but I still want to see him…*
> *F: Is it a bit like parenting…*
> *N: Parents… and leaving home… yes… he's gone through all the stages, I've seen him go through being a teenager behaviour to very mature behaviour*
> *F: And you have known him…?*
> *N: 27 years now…*
> *N: Yes, will be soon, it's just emerged into a very very loving relationship*
> (A. Norah and Bella 2009, December 14)

If not emotional attachment, social continuity was a key concept previously mentioned by Bernard (above). The particular value which a chaplain brought to his advocacy is in saying things which other team members had not realised, Bernard argued:

> *And so I can say things about them which perhaps they hadn't realised, about their background, and sometimes I think it's about issues which they don't think are being addressed, especially as a chaplain, I suppose: spiritual, religious or cultural things which often they feel is being dismissed* [sic]. (Bernard 2008, August 19)

In putting forward issues that the patient did not think were being addressed or *'dismissed,'* particularly in spiritual and cultural areas, and by being with him, he hoped that the individuals would be more confident and empowered to ask questions next time round. This stance fitted in with the previously evoked model of RE since patients or clients were supported in their issues and then, having achieved autonomy based on the recognition of an equal status, were seen to go on to advocate for themselves.

In the discussion I used the description 'self-advocacy' to capture this person-centred approach Bernard and other chaplains were using. In this discussion of empowerment in a spiritual domain there was a lack of information from my data drawn directly from clients themselves. For example, in exploration of the subject with Louise and others:

> *Facilitator: ... How has self-advocacy helped you or other people with services, housing, leisure activities or in relation to god, spirituality*
> > *Louise: God?*
> *F: Yes, are there any ways in which the advocacy service has helped you*
> *Co-F: ... in accessing*
> *F: accessing*
> *Co-F: ... things, not preaching*
> *(Laughter)*
> *F: Helping you do what you want with religion... you know in the culture group we talked a lot about religion... but maybe we haven't done anything... so what has advocacy done to help you, and what sort of things have you had an advocate involved in...*
> > *Whitney: We go to meetings, we train with the police... been... what else?*
> (Louise et al. 2007, November 23)

Broaching the subject of 'God' or spirituality caused a break in the conversation, much of which could have been mitigated with the exercise of more skill by myself as interviewer. More expert work has been done elsewhere in relation to people with learning disabilities (Swinton 2001), and although no mental health clients were among my participants, there has also been work done in this area (Macmin and Foskett 2004). In a later interview in this study, Scoby and Madonna were, however, pertinently responsive:

> *F: Are there ways in which having an advocate or being part of a self-advocacy group has met your social cultural or spiritual needs. So for example if you wanted to learn about other cultures, or learn about religions, or philosophies*

*or faiths, if that's something you have come across as part of advocacy, and if not
do you think it should or could be?*

*Scoby: … I think lots of people have lots of fights over it… like politics, it
happens but we don't often talk about it, we do sometimes.*

*F: If you are a representative group, is it something which comes up in com-
mittee meetings?*

Scoby: No, I wouldn't say that, no, not a lot… no I don't think it does

Madonna: It might hurt somebody's feelings, you know, if you say something
(Micky et al. 2008, May 14)

Both Scoby and Madonna showed cultural and spiritual sensitivity, and it
would have possibly been profitable to press further with that particular
line of questioning. For all people, of whatever ability, talking personally
about spirituality is difficult, *as I acknowledged at my proposal stage*, and
the fact that these clients were grouped together rather than engaged with
one-to-one may have contributed to a poorer outcome. In this section
I covered some of the social and community implications of advocacy:
increasingly it can be seen that an individualist approach to health and
social care, including advocacy, is inadequate. Clearly, from my interviews, the community ethos of the self-advocacy groups modelled a
more corporately recognisable form of action. As Swinton et al. (2011)
noted in a section on 'Spirituality and Community' and in relation to
an individual with more profound disabilities than any I saw in the self-
advocacy groups and indeed than Norah worked with: 'Spirituality is
something that *we* have together. *I am spiritual because we are*' (Swinton
et al. 2011, p. 14).

6.2   Case Study: Contextualising an Advocate's Use
of Spiritual Skills

Being able to meet the social and emotional needs of a client in a social
context (against the inability to do so lamented by Kevin as an *'utter failure'* of advocacy (5.2)) was prioritised by the citizen advocate Norah. She
took up the story about the number of staff her client had had during
the time she had known her. This is an extract from an unpublished piece
which Norah wrote to a health or social care body:

I have no conflict of interest as I do not work for the Health Authority or the Advocacy office. I take my direction from the relationship, not any agency…
    I work to keep a continuity in her life, something she has not had ever
    In the first 7 years that I have known her she has had 122 people caring for her who she is expected to trust and to go to in trouble and 17 doctors…
(A. Norah 1990)

Bella commented on the nature of the above as a resource:

… it's a brilliant tool when you are advocating for people to say, 'We are the continuity, we are the people around constantly feeding you the information, we are the experts, if you like on that person.' (A. Norah and Bella 2009, December 14)

Emotional connection, empathic support and disinterested continuity[4] appeared to be the themes of the nature of this advocate-client relationship from the point of view of the advocate and, through this, made it more possible to discuss spirituality. Norah explained how she found out that one of her clients was a Roman Catholic but since he was also of dual Asian/white ethnicity, she wanted to introduce him *'to both cultures… not necessarily religious culture but the culture of a Hindu'* (A. Norah and Bella 2009, December 14). Norah had not been able to support her client to go to a Temple because she was looking for a man to take him. (Women were forbidden from attending, according to Norah's contact.) This activity was concerned to support a client to discover and explore cultural and spiritual roots, which were important irrespective of one's ability, and to constitute therefore an Action Based on Equality. As a Roman Catholic herself, Norah described her priest making a pastoral visit:

N: Lawrence was here once when he came and I was really pleased and we were sat at the table eating… He was really pleased to see him, the priest was, you know, and now he always asks about him (A. Norah and Bella 2009, December 14)

---

[4] Characteristics of 'empathic imaginative connectedness… indwelling' (Gammack 2011a) constitute my model of Reconstructed Empowerment.

Norah continued to describe another incident with Lawrence:

> *N: I was at church once and he just got up and lay on the floor in the middle of the aisle...*
> *F: Yes*
> *N: and (laughter) someone came running up the aisle with a cushion and put it under his head*
> *F: That's right, people should be able to do what they want...* (A. Norah and Bella 2009, December 14)

At this point in the discussion, as the facilitator, I was getting involved in a debate about church management. But this stance was an advantage because it led to a discussion on the theology of advocacy. When questioned about the fact that some spiritual training had been considered suspect by her previous manager, Norah offered this account of her own faith as a motivation. I have quoted at some length because I wanted to highlight the vocation of a Christian volunteer advocate and touch on another response to SQ1:

> *N: Well, yes, it was, because I was just thinking... especially the Beatitudes, you know... the Beatitudes, you know, and I was talking to another advocate and we were just thinking: 'This is what we do, especially at the beginning, it's the one, you know, 'Feed the hungry...* [5]
> *B: I didn't know what they were, to be honest, I told you, I'm a heathen...*

---

[5] The 'Beatitudes' comprise the teaching of Christ from the Sermon on the Mount: .../...

Blessed are the poor in spirit, for theirs is the kingdom of heaven. Blessed are they who mourn, for they shall be comforted. Blessed are the meek, for they shall inherit the earth. Blessed are they who hunger and thirst for righteousness, for they shall be satisfied.
Matthew 5:3–10 (Bible).

This can be confused with the Parable of the Final Judgement from later in Matthew's gospel:

34 'Then the King will say to those on his right, 'Come, you who are blessed by my Father; take your inheritance, the kingdom prepared for you since the creation of the world. 35 For I was hungry and you gave me something to eat, I was thirsty and you gave me something to drink, I was a stranger and you invited me in, 36 I needed clothes and you clothed me, I was sick and you looked after me, I was in prison and you came to visit me.'
Matthew 25: 34–40 (Bible)

However, in Catholic tradition the 'Seven Corporal Works of Mercy' are based on this text and were likely in Norah's mind (Delany 1911).

N: It's just, everything, 'Give a home to the homeless, feed the hungry…' and it's like all of those were lacking in Lawrence's life… and that most of them through my intervention he has now so that I thought that all these years that I have been a Catholic… and I've always gone to church, I went to a Catholic school, and it didn't really mean that I was really practising my religion until I met Lawrence… it just made it all just fall into place…

B: I'm just surprised really that it just ever seems to be how you are brought up to be… (A. Norah and Bella 2009, December 14)

There was a danger in reading too much into the client Lawrence's faith, from what Norah said about it; as stated above, a more expert assessment could be made. But it was at least clear that for Norah, who supported Kevin socially and culturally, the place of faith was a motivating factor:

N: I didn't do it for the religious reason but afterwards I realised that it was, it could be like that, the basis… maybe had I not had the background I had I wouldn't be (doing advocacy). (A. Norah and Bella 2009, December 14)

6.3   Instructed Advocacy Is Deeply Informed by the Spiritual/Cultural Interface

In differentiation from spiritual care coordinators, and perhaps from Norah as a citizen advocate (rather than a paid employee) with her spiritual motivation above, other advocates generally felt that they would only address spiritual needs indirectly; in other words, the approach to spirituality would need to be instructed and clearly client-led. Angela gave the example of a Muslim client in an acute psychiatric ward:

Taking the question of meeting the spiritual needs of a client, if a client should have those needs it would certainly be our aim to have those needs met, for example there was an acute ward where the spiritual needs of someone going through Ramadan were not being addressed and the advocacy service was able to raise those needs, for instance dietary requirements, and to draw these to the attention of staff. (Angela 2007, October 1)

Although there was no discussion with Angela about the dynamic of spiritual needs, as she said she had had no training in the area, hers was a pragmatic response to the possibility that an individual might not be having their needs met during Ramadan and how an advocate could assist with that. In some ways the advocacy principle of Action Based on Equality was manifested in this concern, not to proselytise, but to meet the spiritual needs as they arose, if they did, in contrast to the role of chaplains, for whom the spiritual dimension was always relevant. Sam mentioned working with a client of dual heritage in a British city:

> *His father was Pakistani but he hadn't had any contact with his father since he was born. He expressed a wish to explore his religious/cultural side of his Asian Pakistani heritage. To begin with he said, well I downloaded some information about different religions, and went through it with him, read through it with him because he wasn't able to read very much himself, and he then decided that he would like to explore Hinduism so I found out where the Hindu temple was in Glasgow and arranged to go along with the client on the Sunday when they had a service. He then decided he actually wanted to be a Muslim so again I found out where the central mosque was... and went there on a number of occasions.* (Sam 2008, February 13)

By contrast, for Sam, researching and discussing religious options with her client, going with the client to a Hindu temple and then to a Mosque and continuing to dialogue about the choices represented a sympathetic form of accompaniment and an expression of Reconstructed Empowerment and Action Based on Equality.

Maria also gave an example of a patient who was street preaching (c. 2002), for whom this was seen as a form of mental disorder. The man, who was in the intensive care unit, had chosen

> *to stand in the middle of the road and preach, that was what he wanted to do, that was his calling, and yet they perceived it as an issue to do with his mental health. And yet people do go and preach in public, don't they, and they can get sent to criminal courts rather than (psychiatric hospital). He thought it was important as a form of witness to spread the news... and this was deemed to be part of his illness...* (Maria 2007, October 1)

Maria observed that the behaviour was considered to be part of the patient's diagnosis and implied that a more comprehensive view would not necessarily see this as the case. This example would need to be set alongside some of the experiences which chaplains noted, as we shall see below. By way of another example, consider again Sam, who worked with refugees who had fled across the South China Sea, and had learnt their 'cultural and spiritual language':

> *One of the organizations I worked with was an organisation called the [name of organisation] which was set up specifically to support clients and service providers to prevent cultural misunderstandings which were leading to huge numbers of misdiagnosed psychiatric illnesses amongst the Chinese and Vietnamese refugees.* (Sam 2008, February 13)

She noted that when they talked of ghosts and conversations with the dead, some were misdiagnosed as having schizophrenia. In fact, professionals had been unaware of a tradition that a Chinese household (from Vietnam) appoints a separate room for the 'ghosts' of the family's ancestors to inhabit and in which 'communion' with these ghosts can take place (Sam 2008, February 13). Specific cultural knowledge and behaviour can improve understanding amongst clients and be spread by advocates: a Muslim advocate, who wore a traditional beard and clothing, explained his method in relation to community and hospital work:

> *H: When it comes to the community they might prefer someone from their own religion so the same background is very important… ethnicity might make a difference, I have experienced that in hospital, even though they have mental health problems they may prefer someone from their own religious background… Jana and I go to the wards together, some people approach her and others approach me; if they have religious beliefs, Muslim people might just approach me…* (Habib 2007, October 1)

Cultural and religious signifiers were an important part of the way an advocate could be effective. Sam had said that as an advocate *'the way you dress is really important'*; she in this case warned against being over-smart as many clients already have too many people dressed in suits and ties in their care *'who are generally people who don't do what (clients) want them to'* (Sam 2008, February 13). This stance is intended to have equalising and empowering force and, in the light of the examples above, is illustrative of Action Based on Equality and RE in Sam's case. Choosing certain cultural religious symbols may make communication more difficult as well as being facilitative of discussion, as Fauzia showed:

> *F: There was an in-patient who saw me, with my headscarf, and when he saw he lost it, he called me a terrorist, the whole lot. I was just passing, it was not relevant...* (Fauzia 2007, October 1)

Being called a *'terrorist'* by a patient/bystander on a ward could be distressing and would, with any possible physical danger, call for a risk assessment to be done by the particular advocacy service or employee. In relation to the above and a previous comment made by the advocate Sam about the advisability of dressing informally, Sarah, as an ordained minister, said that wearing her formal dog collar provided short-cuts for the spiritual conversation she sought to have with patients:

> *I was on a year's contract I was covering for someone else and I thought I've got a year and I know I can spend my time explaining what a chaplain does but actually if you've got a collar on it does it all... see the collar they are more likely to bring up their religious beliefs, and so I am doing a lot more religious stuff, spiritual stuff as well...* (Sarah and Karim 2008, December 4)

In yet another example of meeting spiritual needs, a Christian chaplain was told how he had not prayed hard enough; Zablon took up the story:

> *And then she said, 'I only called you here to pray for me, I didn't think you were coming.' And I said, 'Well, we can't just pray we have got to talk.'... And then she said, 'Your prayer is not strong enough, can you pray a little bit more, with some strength...' 'Yes, I said, I will do that.' And I did that. It was quite interesting. And at the end of it, she said to me, 'You are losing your faith, aren't you?' She saw the difficulty there is of praying in a hospital rather than a church. So I said, 'Probably you are right.' Then I stood by, after she had gone, and then she came back and said, 'Thank you very much.' So I saw both sides of allowing her to talk and also offering prayer. And it was useful for her because she was going through lots of difficulty and just praying and thinking that magically the prayers would just take this away is not quite true. And sometimes we talk about what is happening and then we pray about it, that's what I do anyway.* (Zablon 2008, September 19)

Zablon felt that this was because a certain kind of spirituality was seen by the patient to require a loud praying voice; the chaplain was more interested to talk with the client and felt slightly uncomfortable to pray on a ward rather than in a church or chapel, but this reluctance had a therapeutic intention because the prayers, although considered real by both parties, were contextualised by the chaplain ascertaining a rapport with the patient. This sort of interaction went beyond the role which any advocate could traditionally offer but provided an example of successful communication.

In meeting general cultural or community needs rather than their own needs, advocacy clients or self-advocates themselves reported, as we saw above, about a training session they had led to raise awareness of discrimination with the police (Louise et al. 2007, November 23); another group related how they had spoken about religion in a 'culture group' as part of self-advocacy (Micky et al. 2008, May 14).

The advocacy role of religious professionals—which was again distinctive from what advocates could do in their role—in being a gatekeeper for individual beliefs could be considered further in relation to issues of personal liberty. This was made clear by three examples from spiritual care coordinators. In a separate case a chaplain mentioned that he was asked to write in a patient's notes that her beliefs were *"consistent with her faith group" ... which somehow helped in that... and her treatment was stopped...'* (Zablon 2008, September 19). In another hospital, a chaplain was asked if an individual had *'genuine religious ideas'* (Dorothy 2008, September 18).

Chaplaincy roles could be related to a limited extent to those of IMCAs, in what these advocates needed to do in establishing the views, preferences, beliefs and values of those without capacity to express them at that particular time, in the non-instructed support they provided. In another example from an advocate, a client needed cultural reassurance he was not 'psychotic' on account of the fact he had been praying to African gods:

R: Well, I have actually helped clients attain their spiritual and social needs. As a black advocate I remember helping a black patient actually explain that he is not... psychotic, he was actually praying to whoever he was praying to – it was African gods... (Ruth 2007, November 21)

Culturally Ruth identified her ethnicity as contributing to the support she offered. For a chaplain religion provided similar cultural capital:

> *I'm an honorary black person so really black people laugh at it, they know I am... European, but I am accepted as being black because of Islam.* (Sarah and Karim 2008, December 4)

An example of the social and spiritual support given by a local church to individuals recovering in the community was produced. In relation to an individual of refugee status, a consultant spoke up positively:

> '*What you've done is give this woman a family'... people in the parish... have supported her incredibly well, and that's made a great deal of difference to her.* (Bernard 2008, August 19)

With regard to spiritual needs, it was not straightforward to separate what were clearly spiritual or theological as opposed to cultural needs. One issue which was common in discussion with both Muslim and Christian participants, both chaplains and some advocates, was the phenomenon of 'possession' in relation to mental health. Fauzia spoke of some training material she had read:

> *People got better... It was because they were being told that it was not them who were going mad, they got better, it was amazing, they made speeches saying, 'We are better...'* (Fauzia 2007, October 1)

The patient above, whom Zablon had preferred to speak with rather than pray with, had told him that she felt she was 'possessed' (Zablon 2008, September 19). Another spiritual care coordinator explained about her work with an individual:

> *And I went to see him and he was very distressed, and really his beliefs, his cultural beliefs were not being taken seriously in any way whatsoever by the psychiatrist, simply because he was being told 'It's purely because you are mentally ill, it's got nothing to do with witchcraft...' but after my meeting with him where I took his beliefs seriously I was able to talk to him and meet him where he was and talk through his faith... 'Have you felt even marginally better since*

you have been here?' 'Yes, I have...' 'So the witches aren't perhaps as powerful as you think they are.'... by meeting him at that cultural and spiritual level rather than it being dismissed and those fears growing and it being nurtured, I think it helped him tremendously... (Sarah and Karim 2008, December 4)

Again, this said more about the practice of spiritual care professionals than advocates, but it represented an example of advocacy practice, in taking cultural views and religious beliefs seriously so that change was effected, and one which an emerging profession would need to take seriously.

More research is needed in the area of possession and has been undertaken in the general field of spirituality and mental health (Coyte et al. 2008; Gilbert 2008). In addition, greater attention was being given to the area of spiritual assessment, a responsibility of all healthcare professionals but one which evidently spiritual care coordinators championed:

One of the questions I asked is because in the guidelines for assessment there is, there are sections about diversity, guiding values, spirituality, religion, culture – and I asked the question; 'Do we know whether these areas of assessment are actually used by professionals?' Because my suspicion is that some people do and some people don't. I've provided workshops about assessing spiritual needs but I really want to do that in a much more organized way. (Bernard 2008, August 19)

These questions, which Bernard wanted to keep on the agenda, were certainly ones which, from the conversations I had, both with advocates and other chaplains, would bear repeating and which could implicitly raise certain standards in advocacy practice if attended to carefully.

Using understandings from theology and philosophy, and with reference to virtue ethics and Critical Realism approaches, which will be developed further, I constructed a model for advocacy. This model encompassed and drew attention to spiritual and theological concerns, with Reconstructed Empowerment and Action Based on Equality as centripetal forces within it; but it did not ignore awareness of the distinctive history and practices of advocacy which were very much situated in the interstices of the secular expression of health and social care in the UK, and which were marked by a sense of professionalisation in the making.

With this in mind, I will now summarise what this chapter has brought to the argument before moving into the final substantive chapter.

7   Conclusion

This book is intended to make up a deficit in spiritual discourse in health and social care (and argue for its prima facie purpose) and specifically to establish links between theology, spirituality and advocacy practice. My purpose is to add to the debate about the professionalisation of advocacy by interrogating the practice within the discipline of Practical Theology, in short, to think 'faithfully' about advocacy. As explained in previous chapters, this project's aim is to look at connections within independent voluntary organisations, between advocacy and PPI and personal, theological and spiritual development, and to hear the influential voices.

There were many angles on which chaplains and advocates had shared aims; it would make sense for there to be more solution-focused dialogue. These interweaving lines of argument in Chaps. 4 and 5 were brought to a head in the final section in which I drew out best practices examples based on the voices of advocates and chaplains in relation to their advocacy skills and used in meeting clients' social, cultural and spiritual support needs. The narrative accounted for needs that each of these individuals had at a particular stage of their own story. Within the discipline of Practical Theology from a Christian tradition, predicated on the story of divine creation, humankind's fall, salvation, resurrection and re-creation, I alluded to features of a more holistic and spiritual approach in advocacy. Thus the categories of Reconstructed Empowerment and Action Based on Equality were my attempts to generalise and make normative what I had drawn from what independent advocates (and others using advocacy skills) do. And furthermore, as for how I then constructed what they (advocates) explain they are doing and reflect on as they do it, 'Deep Advocacy' proved to be a useful description of a critically-applied, faith-neutral spiritual virtue ethic. This is what I aim to develop in Chap. 6.

6

Harmonised Voices: Advocacy Practice in the Context of Virtue and Spirituality

1 Introduction

In this final chapter I synthesise voices from practice (identified in Chaps. 2, 4 and 5) with those from literature, theology and philosophy, which were heard in Chap. 3 (Yin 2006, pp. 13–14). In particular, I give attention to key question 3 (Q3 in Appendix 1), philosophical and theological models which can elucidate understanding and responses to Qs 1 and 2. In other words, what do advocates think about professionalisation, and how is advocacy practice explained by those using its skills, including spiritual carers? Practical Theology is the chosen discipline since it is like a 'lake,' to use Pattison's (2000) analogy about what he preferred to call Pastoral Theology, in which I plumb the spiritual, even theological, waters for currents of independent advocacy (Pattison 2000, p. 227). These were found in mental health nursing, the movements of citizen advocacy and self-advocacy, tides of literature and study covering mental health and spirituality, and, last but not least, in some places in the more recent statutory expression of advocacy in the English and Welsh IMCA and IMHA services. Advocacy touches many areas, from statutory through community to the personal. This title from a book made sense:

© The Author(s) 2017   **181**
G. Morgan, *Independent Advocacy and Spiritual Care*,
DOI 10.1057/978-1-137-53125-4_6

'Advocacy for All!' since many 'of us will at some points in our lives look to the support of someone we trust to help us speak up for ourselves' (Gammack 2011a; Scottish-Independent-Advocacy-Alliance 2010). Much of the theory I have elaborated on so far has also been pragmatic and rooted in appreciative enquiry. Thus, the descriptions, Reconstructed Empowerment and Action Based on Equality, have grown out of praxis and provide a way in to the theological issues I examine. That specific way in which advocates set out to support service-users with the practical necessities of everyday life—housing and health decisions in local Western welfare systems—has coloured the portrait of the intricacies of the practice. And on account of that close involvement I can make connections between the practical expression of advocacy and spiritual and theological roots.

Why am I doing this? I am carrying out this examination of independent advocacy in order to enhance understanding of its professionalisation for practitioners in the context of the history of advocacy. Principally it is so that advocates and, secondly, other professionals (such as chaplains) can be assisted to think more holistically, more culturally and spiritually, about advocacy. From here onwards, therefore, I propose a sharper focus on advocacy theory. Although advocacy is not yet fully developed as a profession and does not have an agreed body of knowledge or, indeed, any current registration (e.g. with the Health Professions Council, which incidentally healthcare chaplaincy also lacks), I propose a normative position, using the inclusive framework of Practical Theology, in relation to cultural and spiritual concerns. I have shown that there are gathering experiences, literature and energy, and for that purpose, voices from the discipline of Professional Studies which demand attention, for example, Koehn (1994) and Eraut (1994, 2000, 2004). Because of the link with the selected comparator profession of mental health spiritual care or chaplaincy (see previous chapters), responses to the voices of advocates and their clients will be harmonised with reactions from chaplains.

Secondly, since developments in spirituality are not limited to chaplaincy and, in particular, have been prominent in the field of nursing, I will refer to a couple of voices from that profession towards the end of the chapter. In the Preface and elsewhere I also question whether advocacy can apply more widely and consider case examples of deficits in social care where certain vulnerable individuals' needs have not been met.

2   Hospitality and Spiritual Responsibility Within Advocacy

There is a parallel narrative related to the involvement of chaplains in the fact-finding content of this book, resulting from reflection on the spiritual history of advocacy set out above. For these reasons a relevant caveat is in order. At first sight independent advocacy did not seem to be compliant with any particular religious or theological interpretation, built as it is on a philosophical and human rights platform which does not clearly reach back to pre-existing philosophical or religious foundations. So, as mentioned in Chap. 1, advocacy apparently arose as a secular occupation which performed a humanistic signposting role and was neutral towards faith on account of its necessarily functional purpose. My argument challenges this by adding extra nuances to advocacy, by looking again at its spiritual, cultural and arguably faith roots in history, at interactions between advocates and clients, and by attributing new dimensions to the professionalisation of the occupation. Also, more articulate expressions of advocacy are now found in IMHA and IMCA practice, in which comprehensive and sometimes complex written reports are provided for NHS and social care decision-makers, and in which cultural and spiritual matters can belong within the assessment. This caused the chaplain Oliver to observe that he would love to be an IMCA and that he had '*a gut feeling that advocates have taken over traditional areas of involvement for chaplains*' (5.1).

The ambiguity in the conversation between standard advocacy and its spiritual roots is a line I tread cautiously and respectfully as an advocate-turned healthcare chaplain, and for these reasons I carefully reflected upon this in Chap. 1. Practical Theology embraces this ambiguity in a discipline which is capable of integrating advocacy and spirituality in the overlap of the spheres of human sciences and theology. The increase in literature on spirituality and mental health, which I have noted in Chap. 1 and Sect. 2.1.6 of Chap. 3, and some spiritual and religious expectations in recent statutory advocacy roles such as the need for IMCAs to consider 'beliefs and values' underlie the juxtaposition of the voices of advocates, and clients, with those of chaplains, and defend explanations which will come out of this chapter.

The advantage of locating advocacy in a spiritual as well as a public and political space assists the occupation, service and profession to recover its hospitable and theological credentials. Wolfensberger (2001a), a Roman Catholic layperson, drew on contemporary writers to expand on an insight from his reading of Acts 4:32–35 (Bible): the practice of 'communality' was a mandate for the normative way of living in earliest Christianity. He argued that if the principle of integration of people with learning disabilities, the 'needy, poor, wounded or dependent,' in a Christian congregation were ignored, it would result in that congregation being 'cut off from the suffering Christ,' which would 'put one's salvation at terrible risk' (Wolfensberger 2001b, pp. 117–8). This aspirational 'communal advocacy' related to the theology of churches where members are receptive to talk of the experience of suffering and where responses to vulnerability are developmental. Wolfensberger recognised this in his involvement with the *l'Arche* community of people with learning disabilities (Vanier 2008). Bretherton (2006) also characterised this interaction as flourishing inspired by care of the dependent (3.1.1.). The explicitly Christian virtues indicated here (including active non-discriminating welcome and hospitality) lead to a more holistic, spiritually committed approach to advocacy, which chaplains can also adopt. Practical Theologian Stanley Hauerwas (Hauerwas and Berkman 2005) pertinently referred to the 'hospital' as 'first and foremost a house of hospitality along the way of our journey with finitude'; in the place of 'hospital' one may substitute 'social care' or the 'advocacy service.' In addition, he wanted to avoid linking medicine with 'theological presuppositions.' I am similarly reluctant with advocacy. Given the particular demands put on those who care, Hauerwas indicated that something like a church, even though it will realistically be imperfect, 'is necessary to sustain that care' or to make available communal advocacy. It is in this context that I will consider what kind of spiritual support, or training, will sustain advocates in the service which they are called to provide (Hauerwas and Berkman 2005, pp. 554, 548). These spiritual connections underlie the interpretative concepts of Reconstructed Empowerment and Action Based on Equality within the argument. Thus the health and social care function of advocacy is creatively and fruitfully enhanced in this faith-based conversation and journey. The field of ethics, and specifically 'virtue ethics,' is where this correspondence can take place. I now want to explore in some detail the origins of this philosophical framework since it will be the means by which I come to a conclusion in responding to Q3, the question of which models should be used to link professionalisation, independent advocacy practice and spiritual care within the process of Practical Theology.

3 How Virtue Ethics Spiritually Impacts Advocacy Practice and Well-Being Theory

In philosophy and classical theology, the basis of virtue ethics in *eudai-monia,* translated as 'happiness' or 'well-being,' has provoked thought. Graham (2010) pinpointed the re-emergence of religion in the multi-disciplinary debate about well-being and new conversational opportunities. She noted that 'there are significant overlaps between philosophical thinking about the good life, particularly regarding virtue ethics, and moral theology' (E. Graham 2010, p. 225). The revival of virtue ethics usefully connected with literature on well-being and called for a more dialogic approach to Christian ethics and discussion within Christianity, as well as within other faith and non-faith-based groups (Garnett et al. cited in Graham 2010, p. 228).[1] The incorporation of virtue ethics is facilitated through the 'under-labouring' function of Critical Realism, a crucial stance since it accommodates the transcendental, spiritual and personal within reasoned argument. A definitional survey is useful at this point.

Deriving from strands in moral philosophy grounded in Aristotle (Aristotle et al. 1976) and interpreted through St. Thomas Aquinas, what came to be described as 'virtue ethics' was the preeminent way of theorising in the ancient world. In the last 30 years it was revived by Macintyre and others (MacIntyre 1985; Slote 1997, p. 175). This theory based its judgements on the character traits which in ancient Greece were esteemed, such as courage and wisdom.

For Aristotle:

---

[1] 'The revival of virtue ethics in theology… offers a way of reconciling the potential conflict between law and grace, while indicating such a framework in the public domain… This takes us into… how questions of value and how notions of the good can be negotiated… Can religion be taken seriously as a well-spring of public values, or is it to be seen purely as a sectional, fiduciary [mg.: holding something in trust] language only for the faithful?' (E. Graham 2010, p. 228, [my brackets])

The student of virtue must develop the right habits, so that he tends to perform virtuous acts... although habituation is a tool for character development, it is not equivalent to virtue; virtue requires conscious choice and affirmation. (Athanassoulis 2006).

Thus virtue lay in a mean between two extremes so that, for example, 'patience' (*praotes*) was achieved in an individual who could balance between the excess of 'irascibility' (*ogilotes*) and the deficiency of 'lack of spirit' (*aorgesia*) to get results. Similarly, 'courage' was poised between 'rashness' and 'cowardice,' and classically Aristotle distinguished risk-aware courage, which a good person attained, from the recklessness of the more ancient Greek warrior (Aristotle et al. 1976, pp. 1116a15–1117a29). Thus this was not a counsel of 'moderation in all things' because assertiveness was not ruled out by the need, say, for 'righteous indignation' (placed between 'envy' and 'malicious enjoyment'). The mean lay in what was contextually appropriate to the individual and the situation (Aristotle et al. 1976, p. 104).

Although retrospectively obvious, it was not clear in the first part of the twentieth century how virtue ethics could link with spirituality, and much work was done by Macintyre and his philosophical antecedents in facilitating this turn. The above 'doctrine of the mean' derived from Aristotle's concept of *eudaimonia* (Gr.), as happiness or, literally as 'having a good guardian spirit,' was contaminated definitionally by some philosophers in the 1950s. They misattributed the notion with utilitarian (results-based) or even hedonistic notions of the good life (Aristotle et al. 1976, Book One). This was contrary to *true* Aristotelianism which should have concerned elements which build character to achieve that human goal. This is seen in terms of a more duty-based, or deontological, ethic.

Anscombe (Anscombe 1981) lined up with the latter argument whereas Williams (B. Williams 1985) and Nussbaum (Nussbaum 1986) embraced a deformed version of virtue: they mistook rejection of a Kantian duty-based approach as coterminous with Christian ethics as in Roman Catholic moral theology. This was in some ways understandable as the austerities of law, rules and obedience consonant with Aquinas seemed to exclude more cheering emphases on 'happiness, character, reason' and virtue. (Kerr 2002, pp. 115–6).

From the 1970s onwards, however, some thinkers drew attention to the rehabilitation of a neo-Aristotelian doctrine of natural teleology (contrary to Williams (1985) and Nussbaum (1986)), arguing that it was manifest and unvanquishably inherent in human nature so that virtues of faith, hope, charity, prudence and temperance could not be ignored (Boyle 1982; Geach 1977; Jordan 1986):

> Thomas' (Aquinas) moral theology… is founded not on God's law (biblically revealed or built into creaturely nature) but focused on God's promise of perfect beatitude (revealed by Christ but best understood as the divinely given fulfilment of an Aristotelian conception of human flourishing). (Kerr 2002, p. 118)

Aquinas moved forward to revalorise what then became 'Christian virtues,' namely, notions of humility, which were not placed among the virtues by Aristotle, as Macintyre (1985) pointed out (MacIntyre 1985, p. 136). A neo-Aristotelian, he also believed that these recovered virtues were linked with ulterior well-being and were grounded in, and grew out of, social and political changes, for in 'Whose Justice? Which Rationality?' (1988), he defined justice as

> …that form of life within which to the greatest possible degree the goods of each practice could be enjoyed as well as those goods which are the external rewards of excellence. The name given by Greeks to this form of activity was 'politics,' the polis was the institution whose concern… was with desert and achievement as such… to be eudaimōn… (and to make) a judgement as to what way of life is best and what human flourishing consists in. (K. Knight 1998, p. 112; MacIntyre 1988)

The antidote to injustice and unhappiness was to rediscover a morally coherent discourse in a 'more or less unified moral tradition in which ideals of virtue' play a central role. This led in a structured manner to the thought of the previously cited Hauerwas for whom virtue and character meant more than moral rules in considering the Christian moral life, and whom I consider further below (Porter 2001, p. 98). Equally, another view is that while aiding deliberation on the human telos (purpose) and *eudaimonia* in a more realistic way, virtue ethics would not ask what a virtuous person would do but rather what could be the universal principles (being duty-based) or what could maximise utility (being results-based). It can enable the exploration, in an open-ended way, of the place in life of ideas of well-being and excellence—in other words, what human beings think, think they think or think they had better not think (self-censored discrimination). This enriched 'philosophy of psychology' (Chappell 2013, p. 169) facilitated the study of virtues, vices, emotions and pleasures (Russell 2013). In this book I am referring to the former 'spiritually bounded approach' since the study resides in the discipline of Practical Theology. But the latter more liberal and articulated approach also nests suitably within the Critical Realist container in which I consider closely the professionalisation of advocacy in the voices of different actors, whether they are theologically accented or not.

Thus, virtue ethics can be understood as a process of systematic, critical reflection on the virtues which are likely to emerge in conditions of social change, when received traditions of these virtues undergo development (Gill 2001; Porter 2001, p. 87). Christian thinkers pointed to certain character traits and built on courage and wisdom in a definition of virtues within a Christian virtue tradition as against other virtue traditions. An objection to Roman Catholic and Thomist moral theology was related to the primacy of 'beatitude' within that system. Kant objected that a focus on happiness (*Glückseligkeitslehre*—German: well-being/happiness theory) led one away from the demands of duty into 'egoism' and the desires of individuals (Kerr 2002, pp. 130–131). Kerr (2002) interpreted Aquinas' theological project with its focus on *beatitudo* (Latin: blessedness, happiness) as the 'key to the connection between the doctrine of God, theological ethics and Christology' (a branch of theology dealing with the person, nature and role of Jesus of Nazareth [as Christ, or divinely chosen]). Kerr thought that Aquinas' transformation of Aristotle's notion of happiness, in becoming god-like by understanding the world, held up better as the personally anticipated 'blessedness of face-face vision of God in heaven.' (From the 'beatitudes' of the Christian bible, 'Blessed are the pure in heart, for they will see God' [Matthew 5:8, Bible].) 'Moral considerations in the thought of Aquinas should be seen less as virtue ethics or divine command ethics, but as an ethics of divine beatitude' (Kerr, pp. 130–133). This perception of the emphasis on well-being, rather than on reason or law alone, for the emergence of virtue ethics is key to the way I explore a spiritual approach to advocacy.

The influential philosopher Rawls, whom Macintyre engaged with, also had views on happiness and well-being. Providing in 'The Law of Peoples' (Rawls 1999) a strong argument for the American approach to religion, Rawls cited the later writings of Kant in their presentation of a 'realistic utopia' in which 'all liberal and decent peoples may belong.' He stated further that such a reality would be inimical to 'fundamentalists' for whom it would be a 'nightmare of social fragmentation and false doctrines' (Rawls 1999, p. 126).

> Political liberalism is a liberalism of freedom – in this it stands with Kant, Hegel, and J.S. Mill. (6) It upholds the equal freedom both of liberal and decent peoples and of liberal peoples' free and equal citizens; and it looks to ensure these citizens adequate all-purpose means (primary goods) so that they can make intelligent use of their freedoms. Their spiritual well-being, though, is not guaranteed. Political liberalism does not dismiss spiritual questions as unimportant, but to the contrary, because of their importance, it leaves them for each citizen to decide for himself or herself. This is not to say that religion is somehow 'privatised'; instead it is not 'politicised' (that is, perverted and diminished for ideological ends). (Rawls 1999, p. 127)

Prior to the position above, in 'Theory of Justice' (Rawls 1971), Rawls had outlined his well-known principles which, in relation to the freedom of the individual in equal basic liberties, were firstly expressed most simply in the dictum: 'Do as you would be done by.' The secondary egalitarian difference principle (social and economic inequalities being arranged so that they benefit the most disadvantaged) could be related as a justification for the provision enshrined in the British welfare state and the NHS, being typically available 'free at the point of need.' On the one hand, this neutrality of view could be seen to be in keeping with the rights-based ethos undergirding the development of statutory advocacy in the National Health Service.

It was significant therefore that spiritual well-being was an aspect of personal liberty that Rawls later did not wish to guarantee, for, on the other hand, this American approach to religion seems to be at odds with the whole systems approach to spiritual care within the state-driven NHS in the UK. Incidentally this is also a reason why Wolfensberger's analysis, a US citizen himself, may not always be wholly relevant to the UK scene. Since advocates themselves have no direct responsibility beyond signposting in relation to spiritual matters, it will be illuminating to explore ways in which advocates and chaplains felt that they safeguarded spiritual well-being. This issue belonged to Q3 (what models to use to respond to Q1 and Q2?) and was addressed in. It can also relate helpfully to how social responsibility could grow in certain communities where the most vulnerable were betrayed (see the Preface). However, the rejection of non-politicised religion or spirituality (following Rawls) appears not to provide much protection for vulnerable individuals, who have 'spiritual rights.' If you cannot at all times decide for yourself on 'spiritual questions,' in the light of issues of capacity and consent in certain decisions, (upon which other [professional] people give value to your cognition, and if the non-medical best interests process I have outlined is open to interpretation), the road is clear for a fresh theological apprehension of the role of advocacy.

Virtue (or divine beatitude) ethics and evidence from the interview material of Chaps. 3 and 4, as well as material from Christian texts, combine to assist with a vision of what spiritual rights may consist in. These may be in turn a respectful antidote or balance to the correctly humanistic talk of rights in advocacy: what could either be construed as rule-based or individualistic approaches can be recast into more transcendental or community-related frameworks for action or initiative.

3.1   From Trust, Empathy and Love to 'Spiritual Rights'

Therefore, before I explore Christian thought on the virtues of faith, hope and charity, or 'love,' firstly I consider the human side to faith—namely, how and why you value or place trust in an individual, respecting their dignity. 'Compassion, care, dignity and respect' remain intrinsic to the ideology of the NHS (Singh et al. 2013) and extend through human to spiritual rights. These rights depend on trustful and even covenantal relationship, bringing together the one who is empowered with the one who (re-)constructs that empowerment. Above, I identified trust as an advocacy quality (4.2 (a)). The converse is that sensitivity to disempowerment and to indignity and disrespect calls for action, or Action Based on Equality. Early expressions of independent advocacy were formed on the anvil of recognition that inhumanity and indignity towards individuals based on their mental ill health or disability were unacceptable. In the account of the development of Bethlem Hospital I showed that revulsion towards the undignified exhibition of 'lunatics' (3.1 (b.)) was a stage on the way to the exemplary activism of St. Vincent de Paul in France and later William Tuke, the Quaker, in England. Also, figures such as Jean-Baptiste Pussin and John Perceval, seen as a pioneer of the advocacy movement (1840), harnessed their personal experiences and energies to encourage their hearers to put themselves 'in the place of those... suffering' (Brandon 2007). This illustrated thought and action which were founded on empathy (see 4.1 (c);), love and a sense of equality and religious, often specifically Christian, responsibility, when culturally appropriate. Again, these can be distilled as Action Based on Equality. This compassionate concern with a campaigning edge contributed substantively to some reforms in the 'lunacy laws' in England. Although few participants in my contemporary interviews described themselves explicitly as motivated by spiritual or Christian values, and this was not directly interrogated, it was via virtue ethics itself that moral (not necessarily only spiritual) appeal broadened out. Kevin spoke of advocacy as what one does for one's neighbour, Sam spoke of being an 'equaliser' and Norah of being inspired by the Parable of the Final Judgement (Matthew 25: 25–40) in her approach to advocacy: *It's just everything. 'Give a home to the homeless, feed the hungry...'*

Despite the historical continuum of civil, political and social rights, to which I drew attention in Chap. 3, and the location of independent advocacy as an emerging movement in the early days, there were nonetheless contemporary examples of violations of individual (and institutional) human rights in the experience of advocates, which required addressing. Nebi referred above to the role of peer advocates in challenging victims of institutional abuse (see 4.1. (d) (iii)). In the initial case studies of Chap. 2, I detailed experiences of advocates and chaplains in their encounter with disability discrimination in acute care, the problem of double or triple disadvantage (if a client was from a minority culture where mental health was stigmatised), and the way that advocates support clients in questioning their psychiatric treatment, which would otherwise be imposed upon them. These actions—in accordance with Action Based on Equality—were based on principles of the Disability Discrimination and Mental Capacity Acts, but were also derived from fundamental humanitarian and spiritual impulses. The basis of contemporary advocacy in human rights consciousness was brought out in Chaps. 3 and 4, in the self-advocacy agenda as it grew out of a social movement.

I highlighted distinctive voices linked with the inception of advocacy: on the one hand, it was seen as arising in the 1970s and in the postmodern context of deinstitutionalisation, social rights and political activism. (Traustadóttir 2006; Thompson 2008). A longer view, I maintained and argued elsewhere (Morgan 2010), builds upon the spiritual concerns of early mental health reformers, such as Pinel and Perceval, and applies these to a history of independent advocacy. This can also be considered in liberational theological terms, as a 'preferential option' for the oppressed, if not for the poor (Pattison 1994). In particular, the Department of Health's asserted 'new profession' of IMCA advocates (Dept.-of-Health 2008a) included the statutory responsibility to take into account 'any beliefs and values (e.g. religious, cultural, moral or political) that would be likely to influence the decision in question' (Dept.-for-Constitutional-Affairs 2006b, pp. 20, 65), in accordance with the 'best interests' of a client. All this is consonant with the Human Rights Act framework (specifically, Article Nine: Freedom of Conscience [Thought and Religion]) and the fact that public authorities uphold rights to 'manifest one's religion and beliefs' (Dept.-for-Constitutional-Affairs 2006), both of which locate a conduit for these principles to apply to independent advocacy.

This argument connects the continuing debate about keeping spiritual care, despite the perceived privileged heritage of formal chaplaincy, in the public square with, contrary to this, a right that spiritual care should be available to every individual of whatever belief or not. Thus I built up evidence for the prefiguration of spiritual rights through creative listening to a harmony of voices. Alongside this, relatedly I recognised resistance to the specific threat facing spiritual care/chaplaincy as it relies upon the funding of the state through the National Health Service. For this particular study, willingness by the devout participants and spiritual care coordinators to be interviewed, as well as others who may have personally described themselves as atheists or humanists, can be contrasted with the stance of the National Secular Society which questioned whether the NHS should fund chaplaincy (BBC-News 2009, April 8; Gammell 2009, Feb. 7; see also the medical ethicist Sokol 2009, who argued for the value of chaplaincy). This stance could be viewed as a specific northern or western global cultural problem when large parts of the sub-Saharan and Islamic world, and parts of UK inner cities, depend culturally on spirituality or religion as part of a way of life (Foskett et al. 2004a; Gilbert and Nicholls 2003). In addition, at the time of writing the most recent NHS Chaplaincy Guidelines 2015 are clearer on the responsibility which lies with chaplaincy managers to ensure delivery of 'spiritual care to those whose beliefs are not spiritual in nature' (Swift et al. 2015). Advocacy, from a different 'equality and diversity' heritage, by contrast, although it also had significant funding challenges, was in some ways politically and legally on the ascendant, as I showed above (5.4), in the light of Mental Capacity and Mental Health Acts. But I move on to complete the argument below that advocacy needed to learn from classical disciplines and practices such as theology, chaplaincy and aspects of nursing (see 6.4.2. below and Morgan 2011b). Equally and relatedly, chaplaincy or spiritual care can to be seen as something which an individual had a right to access from a public provider, and, indeed, chaplains and spiritual care coordinators, as well as nurses, often had advocacy-type roles to play, and so the synergy between the occupations was usefully examined through this parallel.

In the UK in early 2012, and with the foresight that the Conservative-Liberal Democrat government would later successfully introduce a policy-defining Health and Social Care Act (despite problems of implementation), the British Prime Minister was heard to say that he wanted more 'patient-led visits.' In the course of preparing the background for this book from 2005, I have already drawn attention to some changes in policy. In the next sub-section I will differentiate aspects of the patient-led and self-advocacy movements according to the principles of spiritual rights and virtues.

3.2   Social Movements, Patient-Led Services, Self-Advocacy and Spiritual Virtues

Comparative historical accounts of advocacy in different contexts including Austria, the Netherlands and Sweden, showed how people with learning disabilities became self-advocates and took increasing control of their own lives from the late 1960s onwards. These were influential factors in the emergence of service-based advocacy, as I wondered to what extent advocacy and PPI could be viewed as social or 'prefigurative' movements (see Chap. 3 Sect. 2.1.6. and footnote 3). The examples of Yolanda standing up for herself at work and Dorothy's interrogation of the use of advocates were both examples, respectively, of Reconstructed Empowerment and Action Based on Equality. For Yolanda, a strong consciousness of equal rights and her self-empowerment improved her status at work in relation to the individual who allegedly bullied her. Whether he had a learning disability or not, her self-advocacy had a favourable outcome. Wolfensberger himself did not favour 'self-advocacy,' believing that this detracted from true 'selfless' advocacy and that self-denial rather than self-preservation was the better way. However, a rights-based approach does not contradict the responsibility which Yolanda showed, a balanced righteous confidence consonant with the Aristotelian mean, which protected her own position without recourse to the advocacy of others.

In the case of the chaplain Dorothy's observation that the advocate's actions made staff feel that the patients have more rights than they do, this may indicate that the advocate was attending successfully to equality-promoting action in the work being done (5.2.). Participants (Michael and Micky) made clear the difference between advocacy and self-advocacy; for them advocacy represented a one-to-one relationship, but self-advocacy was a group process: doing *things together,*' as they were empowered. I made reference to 'well-being' and a discussion of the meaning of empowerment (4.3.1.). Duncan (2002) made references to empowerment as ephemeral when applied to statutory transfers of power, a form of lip service to public involvement. This genre of criticism increased in a period of economic austerity (from 2010), in which the 'Big Society' plank in the UK's coalition government policy was seen as leading to an increase in volunteering in inverse proportion to cost-cutting (Duncan 2002). In addition, Fielding (1996) asked how we can help others to feel empowered when we are using our own authority and privilege to do so (Fielding 1996). This is related to a point Kevin (Kevin 2008, January 14) made about the failure of advocacy services because, despite work with some clients for a long period of time, *'their community connections, their kinship, their friendships were no stronger'* (5.3.). For these reasons the need for a more comprehensive model of empowerment was necessary. This is why the emergence of the theme of Reconstructed Empowerment helps to reconstitute the function of advocacy in relation to well-being. A spiritual and theological interpretation of Reconstructed Empowerment can draw on the biblical virtues of faith, hope and love, which provide impetus in securing one's own rights, as well as those of others (see 6.3.5. below).

In reflecting more on well-being and virtue, in the next section I turn to the theological impact of the exercise of qualities and virtues, which I have previously drawn out from participants as being particularly associated with advocacy. This helps with a move towards a 'theology of advocacy.'

3.3 How Deep Advocacy Implies Sacrifice and Struggle

Above I discussed the essential qualities for advocates and their interface with Aristotelian and, later, Christian (St. Paul's) virtues. I noted in the literature review that Wolfensberger, a founding father of advocacy, believed it was not enough to speak on behalf of another, but that advocacy, in his words, implied 'a vigor, a vehemence, a commitment,... a high cost, often in the form of risk,' which could lead to 'hostility from others, taunts, being considered foolish or crazy, loss of income, loss of job, loss of health, physical hurt and violence – perhaps even of death' (see Sect. 3 of Chap. 3). These calls to commitment have parallels in Judeo-Christian and Islamic traditions, for example, Christ's call to his followers to 'Forsake all and follow him' (Mark 10: 17–31, Bible) to be authentically Christian. Equally, the Pillars of Wisdom in Islam enjoin Muslims to a costly rhythm of prayer, fasting and pilgrimage related to a theme of struggle (*jihad*). Aquinas extended the discussion of the virtue of courage or 'fortitude' based on Aristotle, who said it was proven on the battlefield alone, to include exposure to other risks, such as infection or fear of shipwreck, or robbers. Hauerwas (Hauerwas and Berkman 2005) went on to suggest that Aquinas was referring to the missionary journeys of St. Paul or the Parable of the Good Samaritan with these allusions. In fact, the rhetoric of St. Paul when he boasts of his sufferings—'Three times I was beaten with rods, once I was stoned, three times I was shipwrecked… I have been constantly on the move…' (2 Corinthians 11: 25–26, Bible)—can be associated with the passion with which Wolfensberger expressed himself concerning the advocate's inner striving and its outward expression. Further development of Wolfensberger's thought would be useful, based on his past as part of a war-time Jewish community which emigrated from Germany, but there is not space here for a fuller critique of his views (see Gammack 2011a, p. 264; Gaventa and Coulter 2001; Hauerwas and Berkman 2005, pp. 298–299).

The sacrificial aspect of this call to 'deep advocacy,' which I have highlighted and which may not be sufficiently captured in self-advocacy, illustrated an aspect of the reconstruction of empowerment (Reconstructed Empowerment). The desired enthusiasm and commitment of advocates, especially a willingness to give freely of one's time (e.g. to be a volunteer) could be linked with the attitudes of my participants. Bella stated that she did not find advocacy '*easy*' and learnt from volunteers. This could be described as an ethically virtuous stance, noting that Bella differentiated herself from Norah by not being spiritually motivated. Norah, as a volunteer citizen advocate, remarked, in relation to the independence of the advocacy service, that she would '*not lose her job*' whatever she did. Norah showed her preparedness to take risks—which her organisation equipped her to take—when advocating persistently for her client who was finding it difficult to get treated, as we mentioned above. The chaplain Sarah spoke of how the whole atmosphere changed in a ward round as a result of her advocacy for a client who had been '*spoken at*' and whom staff then began to '*affirm*'; this was a clear example of a development in self-empowerment or Reconstructed Empowerment (see 2.3 (a)).

These examples also demonstrated how the practice concepts of Reconstructed Empowerment and Action Based on Equality are linked. The basis for Norah's and Sarah's interventions were that the individuals had equal rights and were valued by their Creator. One was employed by the NHS; the other was a volunteer. It so happened from the evidence that both these advocates were motivated by Christian commitment and St. Paul's scale of virtues, but the absence of this would not make the effort less spiritual. To take another example, Sam spoke of the advocacy principle of treating people as if they did not have a disability, and these actions, based on equal rights, showed willingness to commit oneself personally as one would do for one's neighbour or brother (Chap 4 Sect. 3.2.4.). The chaplain Karim mentioned an advocate colleague, who had continued to be a point of contact with the ward after disengaging with all clinical staff; he also drew attention to the value of the experience of being a service-user, which some mental health advocates brought to the practice (2.3.3.). All these factors showed a commitment to and passion for equal rights, which was beyond the call of duty, a humanitarian urge (after Wolfensberger) which bordered on, and sometimes became, a spiritual or religious expression heralding transformation. The moment of transformation, which was mentioned above in relation to Sarah's pastoral care and the effect on the client, counted as Reconstructed Empowerment, and the mode of operation she and others engaged in I have classified as Action Based on Equality.

3.4   How Deep Advocacy Includes Competence, Virtue and Universalised Spiritual Well-Being

Returning to the immediate context of advocacy practice, the characters of individual advocates or self-advocates, and of advocacy clients, were socially, culturally and spiritually tested as they encountered the system (5.6.). They carried out actions which were appropriate in the context of the cultural community or the required social rebalancing, as they addressed their practical tasks. Above I referred to the well-boundaried support advocates (including chaplains) give as a subtle 'drawing alongside' and the emotional leverage found in the combined forces of the advocate when accompanying the client, based on powerlessness, honesty and realism (4.3.2.). The extensive references to the role of attitude (as well as skills) to what could not evidently be taught (4.3.1.) but needed nonetheless to be inculcated, were weighed against the demonstrable need for the occupation of advocate to become professionalised with appropriate levels of academic and experiential qualifications. How advocates showed a range of notionally moral or religious virtues and then related to, assented to or challenged the system were relevant to their success insofar as, for example, they either achieved changes or contributed to decision-making or ,indeed, persuaded commissioners to continue to fund their service. The example from the Court of Protection showed how valued advocates can become in public life. The IMCA, who was instructed through the DoLS process, demonstrated nuanced empowerment in that she was there to support the client's father on his way through the courts (Reconstructed Empowerment) as well as to ensure that Steven's best interests (i.e. his chosen path) were safeguarded (Action Based on Equality). I was also conscious how the balancing of virtues and vices, envisaged in Aristotelian ethics, took place in the limited but decisive role which the IMCA DoLS advocate played, and in particular in the way she acquitted herself in the documentary radio programme (see 2.2).

The influential philosopher, with theological sympathies, MacIntyre (1999) argued, as I touched on above, for the virtues of 'acknowledged dependence' in those individuals who lack capacity or those whom advocates work with regularly. In his discussion of the political and social structures of the common good, he seemed incidentally to define aspects of the role of the specialist type of advocate, the '39D DoLS IMCA,' when he outlined the 'proxy's role':

> The proxy's role is to speak for those… disabled both inside and outside the community in just the way that that particular disabled individual would have done so for her or himself, had she or he still been able to speak. (MacIntyre 1999, pp. 139,146)

The fact that the common good—for MacIntyre saw practice as straining towards the production of 'internal goods'—beckons us to be 'practical reasoners,' and to reflect that since in the same way that we were all once dependent children, we may also at some undetermined future time become disabled or 'differently-abled.'[2] Giving and receiving, which are necessary for social flourishing to take place in these circumstances, were related to the virtues of independence and acknowledged dependence which, as Macintyre argued, were to be sought after and used to this end (MacIntyre 1999, p. 139). Moreover, for Wolfensberger (2001a), intrinsic to the good life for the learning disabled was the need for 'communality' or partnership between the 'handicapped' (his outdated, but preferred term) and the advocate to be long-term or in some cases 'life-long.' He saw this very communality as a safety net in the case of the death of 'parents, a guardian (or) a strong citizen advocate' (see also Vanier 2008; Wolfensberger 2001a, pp. 106–7).

The quotation from MacIntyre (1999) can be linked to the earlier definition given in Chap. 1: of advocacy as 'speaking up' for others although it must be stressed that the latter related broadly to instructed advocacy, of the kind which Wolfensberger implied. In using the term 'proxy,' MacIntyre defined the narrower relationship with non-instructed advocacy, such as the IMCA. This mapped on to the practical terminology of Mental Capacity best interests, which was set out in the Act as a checklist and was relevant to the Neary case (discussed above in 2.2). The best interests checklist (e.g. 'Encourage participation... Avoid discrimination... Avoid restricting the person's rights' [(DoH) 2008b pp. 65–66]) was intended to be distinguished from 'medical best interests'. I explained how Dunn et al. (2007) perceived the problems of this 'proxy' or 'substitute decision-making' role. The best interests process had as its aim the resolution of a range of subjective dilemmas using an objective framework, according to these authors, who criticised a lack of guidance in the 'process of determination' (Dunn et al. 2007). These debates were all helpful in answering SQ2—regarding the way professionalisation was affected by discussions about the nature of advocacy practice. This problem could conceivably be avoided with a more fully-orbed best interests checklist which attends socially, culturally, spiritually and therapeutically to the needs of the individual, say, with the deployment of a good citizen advocate or support worker. In this sense 'empowerment'

---

[2] My expression.

can be deliberated upon, passed through philosophical and legal filters, and 'reconstructed.'

Given the background of generic advocacy, the build-up of effective supervised practice in statutory IMCA advocacy and increasing case-law, based on the accumulated background in citizen advocacy, and the virtues sharpened in this practice, I argue that these issues are being addressed, but need sustaining. To provide examples, Angela's advocacy for her friend with mental health problems can be classed as Reconstructed Empowerment; and Norah's defence—as a citizen advocate—of the best interests of her learning disabled 'partner' or 'client,' who was in a hospital with a ruptured artery, in a situation where he would not have been treated but for her intervention, can be viewed as Action Based on Equality. A medical best interests' model would have rejected her client or 'partner' as a potential patient in the hospital although his injuries turned out to have been life-threatening. The invaluable role of non-instructed citizen advocacy as a safeguard, espousing the human rights of the 'unbefriended' and disabled, was clearly demonstrated. Both Angela's and Norah's actions were carried out as humanitarian interventions, as Angela empowered her friend, having pondered carefully what was going on in the relationship with mental health services (Reconstructed Empowerment), and as Norah stood up for the rights of a disabled person in a cost-cutting health service (Action Based on Equality). These were not actions which anyone would do for their neighbour unless they had got to know them extremely well or a service had drawn them to their attention. These were examples of advocacy for which Norah later offered a spiritual rationale:

> It's just, everything, 'Give a home to the homeless, feed the hungry...' and it's like all of those were lacking in Lawrence's life... and that most of them through my intervention he has now. So that I thought that all these years that I have been a Catholic... and I've always gone to church, I went to a Catholic school... and it didn't really mean that I was really practicing my religion until I met Lawrence... it just made it all just fall into place... (A. Norah and Bella 2009, December 14).

In this last example it was spirituality, faith or connection with spiritual care grounded in theology, which gave the advocacy actions extra purchase insofar as the biblical principles of Matthew 25 (or the Seven Corporal Works of Mercy [see footnote 34])were followed. They also implied the presence of virtues (such as friendliness, generosity) in the client and the advocate; the client actually brought something to both advocates—in the first example, a new career path for Angela; in the second, a deepening of faith for both concerned. However, incentives to meet basic healthcare and housing needs (Matthew 25: 34–36, Bible) with social, cultural, emotional and 'compositely' spiritual goods are enshrined in both non-faith and faith ethical positions.

Eudaimonia preceded and informed other virtues such as honour, pleasure or intelligence for 'Happiness… is the end at which all actions aim' (Aristotle et al. 1976, Book 1:vii). Aristotelian ethics mediated through Aquinas were discussed by Hauerwas (Hauerwas and Berkman 2005), with support from MacIntyre (1990). It was chronologically novel, as we saw above, that Aquinas should indicate that natural virtues needed to be directed through the way of faith, hope and love to divine ends. This came as a recognition of humankind's disobedience and as part of his project in reframing theological ethics (Hauerwas and Berkman 2005, p. 41; MacIntyre 1990, p. 140). These terms are crucial Christian terms and embraced in the discipline of Practical Theology. As my argument moves closer to a standard Christian theological position, since I frame my own findings with reference to Christian theological virtues, I take care not to exclude other faiths—for example, taking on board the injunction to give alms in Islam—or those with no faith position, on account of the secular, inclusive and universal function of advocacy. In proposing a new normal, I give some recognition—although without the space fully to discuss it—to the field of Spirituality Studies, in which faith is fluid and non-faith-based or existential spirituality also plays a part (e.g. see Gilbert 2011 and the British Association for the Study of Spirituality and its journal).[3]

Again, from a non-faith position, I referred to Professor Richard Layard, the 'happiness czar.' He commented on the 'Measuring National Well-

---

[3] See also Chap. 1.

Being' report (Office-for-National-Statistics 2012), designed by the UK government to provide an alternative measure of national performance to gross domestic product, since it highlighted 'the main factors that influence wellbeing – in particular, health, disability and mental health' and hoped that it would lead to increased investment (Stephenson 2012).[4] Elsewhere Layard (2007) argued that despite living standards being better than 50 years ago in the UK, people were no happier and expressed his 'hope that the churches will do more to help people train their minds in the mental disciplines which we know can lead to serenity and compassion' (Layard 2007, pp. 2, 13). Related to this, I see that independent advocacy is one approach within health and social care and the community and voluntary sector, which is sometimes funded, and which can address this well-being deficit, a factor in which Layard himself suggested that spirituality or faith can have a role.

Above I gathered together some characteristics of advocates: patience, tenacity, enabling the other to be heard, integrity, ability to safeguard and loving one's neighbour or 'equalising.' If one takes Aristotelian virtues and matches some of them with previously elicited advocacy qualities, certain universal correlations may be deduced. For example, Courage (cf. the ability to safeguard and the challenging roles around Action Based on Equality); Temperance; Liberality/Generosity; Greatness of soul; Proper ambition (cf. Reconstructed Empowerment, in the sense of 'knowing one's place'); Patience/Gentleness (cf. the patience of the advocate); Truthfulness (cf. Action Based on Equality or being level with a client); Wittiness; Friendliness (cf. loving one's neighbour); Righteous Indignation (cf. Action Based on [non-discriminatory] Equality); Modesty (cf. enabling the other to be heard in Reconstructed Empowerment). In Book Six Aristotle differentiates between Prudence (or Practical reasoning) and Wisdom (or Theoretical knowledge). This latter is a helpful distinction for my purpose in linking advocacy practice with a more developed theory (Aristotle et al. 1976).

---

[4] Layard is programme director for well-being at the centre for economic performance at the London School of Economics. He said that a key finding in the report was the fact unhappiness and anxiety cut across factors such as occupation, ethnic background and where people lived. 'One of the key things this tells us is that we need a much wider concept of deprivation beyond economic deprivation,' he said.

Were I to universalise the theory, similarities are also found by triangulating Aristotelian and advocacy qualities with Christian virtues—to take examples from a spiritual tradition—as portrayed in the discourses on the meaning of faith, hope and love, referred to already, namely the 'fruit of the spirit' in St. Paul's letters to the Corinthians and Galatians (1 Corinthians 13; Galatians 5:22, Bible). Patience and tenacity (or faithfulness) constitute features both of Aristotelian and Christian ethical systems. In 4.3.2. (above) I noted the vocation to 'love one's neighbour as oneself' as amongst the essential qualities of advocates from the interviews.[5] Advocates have to be *very patient and let people talk about an issue... until the really important things come to the top'* (Olive 2007, November 7). Although the advocate is not a therapist, this approach indicates some level of pastoral skill which chaplains or spiritual care professionals may be able to pass on usefully.

A modern neo-Aristotelian, and Thomist, approach, represented an alternative to deontological (Kantian, rule-based), consequentialist (situationist or results-based) or utilitarian ethical approaches. This became popular with evident influence in the theological domain (Darwall 2002; MacIntyre 1985; Slote 1997), as it related actions to the character attributes of individual actors. For MacIntyre, 'practice,' with which I have been concerned in relation to advocates, was

> a cooperative activity that has standards of excellence in the pursuit of which 'goods internal' to the practice are realized and human powers to achieve excellence are extended. (MacIntyre cited in Hauerwas 1993, p. 118)

Influenced thus by MacIntyre and others, in 2001 Hauerwas revised his approach to the 'ethics of character' and recognised fresh cooperative dimensions regarding the virtues. For him these now encompassed the metaphors of dialogue, journey and community (especially the Church as a 'storied community') in which to discuss the development of the ethics of character (Hauerwas and Berkman 2005, p. 87). Rather than

---

[5] As well as being the foundational Jewish and Christian injunction (Bible: Deuteronomy 6:4–9; Mark 12:29–30). See further below.

abstract philosophical or theological arguments, Hauerwas wanted to highlight narrative and spiritual progress as key to character formation in the 'Christian community.' Alongside 'dialogue, journey and community' one may point to faith, hope and love as respectively and concretely conducive of this formation. I will develop these themes below. Similar to how Layard has approved well-being measures, the UK government has been encouraging the measurement of care and compassion as a reaction to dissatisfaction and failures in NHS hospital care. Bradshaw (2009) described compassion as often seen to be a subjective experience (and therefore difficult to measure) rather than 'rooted and grounded in the Judaeo-Christian framework… underpinned by the narrative encapsulated in the Good Samaritan.' Amnesia about a prior framework, which some want to address in nursing training, could equally apply to advocacy as it possesses a similarly theologically grounded heritage which is in danger of being forgotten (A. Bradshaw 2009, p. 466).

In the light of what I have previously explored with regard to attitude and advocacy training, Hauerwas spoke on courage, of a 'right "attitude"' that included having the appropriate emotions (requiring) training, for we 'become what we are only through the gradual build-up of the appropriate characteristics' (Hauerwas and Berkman 2005, p. 291). This is entirely consonant with the undervalued classic approaches to nursing indicated by Bradshaw (2009, 2011), which are also derived from Aristotle. As evidenced, critiques and mediations of the Aristotelian approach to virtue have been carried out by many, including MacIntyre and Hauerwas. Others of a more conservative viewpoint have corrected the interpreters for not being more theologically attuned (P.W. Lewis 1998; Northcott 2003; Winston and Tucker 2011). Northcott (2003), for example, applauded the later work, 'Dependent Rational Animals' (MacIntyre 1999) for bringing MacIntyre 'much closer to the "Christian narratives of the good life."' It revised a previous heroic account of the Aristotelian virtues with the 'moral priority of dependence, vulnerability and weakness,' and here Northcott (2003) accused MacIntyre (1999), who was also attributed in the article with a later life conversion to Roman Catholicism, of shying away from the overcoming power of the 'folly of the cross,' for these virtues…

are only knowable for Christians, and realizable in their lives, through their communal and individual shaping by the narratives of Christ crucified and risen, through their celebration of the sacraments, in which Christ is really present to them in their worship, and through the performance of lives which are shaped by the Spirit who is the pro-genitor of what Aquinas called the virtues, what St Paul called the fruit of the Spirit in their lives. (Gal. 5:22–24) (Northcott 2003, p. 550)

This exclusivist and slightly uncomfortable Christian claim to virtue led on to an assertion that without the 'cruciform shape of Christ's life,' Christian communities through history have mostly, but not invariably, shown a greater concern for the disabled, the sick, the poor, the weak than the 'empires' in which those communities were set. Imbibed from his time in Malaysia, Northcott (2003) defined this spiritual and Christian ideal against an Islamic suspicion of a theology of weakness (perhaps found precisely in the beatitudes.) Islamic rejection of aspects of Christian faith history means, for example, that not all Muslims and Christians are likely to share wholly a narrative of vulnerability and weakness, he argued (Northcott 2003, p. 550). It is the virtues, or the 'fruit of the spirit,' from the Christian tradition, if one wishes to identify this as such, which shape 'fall-transcending' communities and potentialities, after Wolfensberger, and which can be applied to advocacy (Wolfensberger 2001a, p. 106) .

Could spiritual and religious community social concern, had it been precisely concretised, offered and provided in their home towns, or perhaps through local agencies or churches (plus opportunities to belong, or communality after Wolfensberger), have protected individuals with learning disabilities as mentioned above, or those in Haut de La Garenne, Jersey, where specifically children's advocacy was called for? (Batty 2008; Naughtie 2008) This community concern also now belongs with the work of chaplains (Cobb 2004; Swift et al. 2015, pp. 20–23) but sits very well with the general objectives of independent advocacy and the dynamics which are described in the concepts of Reconstructed Empowerment and Action Based on Equality. What spiritual virtue ethicists imply is a deconstruction of the human power alone to support and campaign for the rights of the other. It also indicates a spirituality- and faith-based, and, if culturally appropriate, Christian reconstruction of empowerment, whether in the action of a volunteer worker or advocate, remunerated or not. In the next sub-section I suggest how St. Paul's triad of virtues can assist reflection on the advocacy process.

3.5   Virtuous Advocacy Reconstructed in Trust, Hope and Compassion

In an article titled, 'Salvation and Health: why medicine needs the church' (1985), Hauerwas drew attention from the Hebrew Bible to Job's comforters. For him they get a 'bad write-up,' but 'at least they sat on the ground with him seven days' (Job 2:13, Bible). Psychiatrist/theologian Frank Lake, the influential figure from cross-disciplinary training (1.2), pointed to Ezekiel—who was also where the exiles sat 'overwhelmed' for seven days (Ezekiel 3:15, Bible)—to show the need for acceptance and empathy as a starting point in 'dynamic' pastoral encounters. If physicians, nurses, chaplains and, perhaps, advocates (of any or no faith) are 'present to the ill' or the disabled in a distinctive way, and if they are the 'bridge between the world of the ill' or of those with disabilities and the 'world of the healthy,' or of those who have learnt to live triumphantly with an impairment of one kind or another, it will be instructive theologically to consider the resources with which anyone can sit in that place and specifically how an independent advocate can do this. Job's comforters, in the example of Hauerwas (2005), did not relieve suffering or distract attention from it but were simply present in the face of that suffering (Hauerwas and Berkman 2005, p. 551). Any human advocate will not usually have transcendent powers in her or himself, but, again turning to Wolfensberger, within the origin of independent advocacy lies divine 'fall-transcending,' transforming power which can be appropriated and which I would call the 'spirit of advocacy' (Morgan 2014; Wolfensberger 2001a, p. 106). In this way the advocate becomes a bridge in the manner envisaged by Hauerwas.

Throughout this book I have incorporated allusions to the Christian Bible (and other religious texts) as relevant interpretatively to the practice of advocacy (e.g. Christ's Sermon on the Mount or the Parable of the Final Judgement [Matthew 25:34–40]; Matthew 6:4, 7:1; Mark

12:29–30 John 17:11; 1 Corinthians 13; Galatians 5:22; James 1:27; also, above from the Hebrew Bible, Deuteronomy 6: 4–9; Job 2:13 and Ezekiel 3:15). The Revised Standard Version translation of the first epistle of John reads:

> My little children, I am writing this to you so that you may not sin; but if any one does sin, we have an advocate with the Father, Jesus Christ the righteous; and he is the expiation for our sins, and not for ours only but also for the sins of the whole world. (1 John 2:1ff., Bible)

This sentence is memorably incorporated into the Common Worship (and the Book of Common Prayer) of the Church of England Holy Communion service books as part of 'The Comfortable Words' prior to the Eucharistic prayer (the prayer at the moment of the blessing of the symbolic bread). Elsewhere the word 'advocate' (Gk: *parakletos*) is translated as counsellor, comforter or helper. In the New International Version of the Bible, it is rephrased as to 'speak in the defence of' a person. These are all seen as ways to convey the response of 'God' to the vulnerable, the lost, the hopeless or desperate. Lake defined this legalistic dynamic as a 'perilous paraklesis.' This concerned the action of one 'called alongside' to help, who 'accepts the responsible task of keeping the defence moving until it "rests" successfully against all the prosecution can do to destroy our self-esteem...' Jesus of Nazareth, said Lake, first faced this danger fully on our behalf and was identified with the 'sickness unto death' with all its despair, darkness and desolation which are, according to Lake, universal (Lake cited in Gammack 2011a, pp. xi, 52). In what way can this Christological interpretation hold meaning for an advocate who would see herself as entirely non-faith-based or secular? Bradshaw (2009) pointed to the fact that the virtue of compassion in care, which is pertinent to advocacy, has an universalisable moral and intellectual component. Whether or not one could trace the cultivation of virtuous character (which results in effective care in nursing and advocacy) back to the Judaeo-Christian tradition does not necessarily detract from the ontological meaning of advocacy, expressed above, or from the actions which take place in its name. Although this does not place the practice of 'speaking in the defence of a person' in the category of a religious activity, aligning oneself with the other can be loosely interpreted as a neighbourly selfless, even 'Christ-like,' act (A. Bradshaw 2009, p. 466).

Already above, Ruth has stressed (Chap. 4 Sect. 3.2.3.), the need for empathy, to have *an ability to see it from (the) position* of the clients, linked to *a knowledge base of what it is that they are up against.'* In relation to this motif of empathy and trust, there was evidence that an advocate was someone with whom trust was engendered in communication. It was *a person who inspires trust'* (Kevin). I also drew attention (in Sect. 1.1 of Chap. 3) to what I described as an early incarnation of the ombudsman from the Old Norse, *umbodhsmadhr,* which meant a 'trusty manager.' When Janine spoke of being the *'mouthpiece'* of a client and smoothing the communication process, and Angela of how she supported her friend, both illustrated the transparency and directness which contrasted with the poorer experience the clients had of other professionals, as Angela's testimony showed. How can a spiritual and transcendental model of the advocate, a Christological interpretation, help to uncover the deeper roots of advocacy? I want to interpret the three bridging virtues of faith, hope and love from St. Paul in 1 Corinthians 13 to carry this conversation forward.

3.5.1   Trust (Faith), Covenant and Reconstructed Empowerment

According to Northcott (2003), St. Paul called Christians to show the 'fruit of the Spirit' in the worship and performance of their lives, that same Spirit who is the progenitor of the virtues, as Thomas Aquinas put it (see 6.2 above). It also seemed that the core meanings of the theological virtues were most clearly expressed in worship and therefore acquired a dynamic character in promoting 'faith that God is the author of all things; hope that God is restoring all things to their original order to God; and love of God and of God's work because they are revealed as loveable' (Northcott 2003, p. 550). Faith is not a virtue in itself but points to that which is beyond and outside experience, apprehension of, and any relationship with, the divine and transcendental being, if one chooses to accept this.

In relation to faith and trust, in her work, Koehn (1994) firstly highlighted the 'un*trust*worthiness of professional experience' and the limitations of 'delegitimating client contracts' as either grounds or workable frameworks for professional authority. Interestingly, for my argument, in the place of these models, she posited the moral, public pledge or 'covenant' as a basis for professionalisation. And, as an illustration from religious practice, those who keep the covenant (Yahweh's faith in his people) which God made with Abraham, in Koehn's terms, will reap peace on the earth (Koehn 1994, p. 81). The role of trust and, by extension, faith, in a 'covenant'-model as a desirable component in the accepted literature around paradigms of professionalism, is indicative of the part that spirituality, Judaeo-Christian theology, and the narrative of the Hebrew Bible can play. This assists understanding of and conversation about a deeper theological trajectory at work within the advocacy project.

Examples from the case studies in Chap. 2, in which advocates (including chaplains) were shown to combat stigma, cultural barriers and psychiatric opinion, indicated an underlying covenantal approach, one which, according to the Christian Bible injunction, goes the extra mile (Matthew 5:42, Bible), which believes the best in and for people (1 Corinthians: 13:7, Bible; see 2.3.1.-3.). In Sect. 6.1 of Chap. 5 Norah spoke of her passionate support for the client, Lawrence, whose treatment within the system was extremely poor, and how her independence was a strength to him (5.6.2. above). Elsewhere her colleague Bella spoke of the fact that a good (citizen) advocate will be more loyal to her client than to the service for which she works. She said that as a volunteer she felt empowered because there was no one to sack her (4.2.3.).

The unwavering commitment of individual to individual here could be said, at the risk of sounding grandiose, to be related to the unconditional commitment of the Hebrew God to his people in the covenant. This depended on the character formation which the people of Israel received through Abraham and the interactions as part of their story. Gammack (2011a) related advocacy to another Hebrew character, Moses, as he responded actively to the oppression of the people of Israel. In an advocate, the virtues of a whole person as part of their own story, which are meaningful collectively rather than atomistically in an Aristotelian way, and which for the Christian are integrated in the 'fruit of the spirit,' could be seen to be demonstrated in these examples.[6] A covenantal (trust- and rule-based) model of advocacy engagement could thus be used to deconstruct power as it is used by social or healthcare actors with clients, service-users or patients. It can support individual clients to be empowered to reconstruct their own power or, indeed, to equip advocates for professionalisation in their service.

3.5.2　Hope and Action Based on Equality

As well as faith and covenant, hope is a major ingredient of spiritual and Christian life and teaching. It is defined as a patient expectation of God's future, or 'perseverance in faith,' which finds the meaning of the present moment not in itself but in the Holy Other. For Christians, hope expresses a genuine truth about God. God is faithful and our hope, as Barrett (1971) commented. God is seen as one in whom faith and hope properly repose (Barrett 1971, p. 309). For Bruce (1964), the assertion that faith is the 'assurance of things hoped for, the conviction of things not seen' (Hebrews 11:1: Bible), signified that things which have no prior existence become real by the exercise of faith (Bruce 1964, p. 278). In a psychological study, Koenig and Larson (2001) pointed to levels of positive association appearing as hope, optimism, purpose and meaning amongst 'religious people.' Not a single study showed that the religious had less hope or optimism than the non-religious. They also found that meaning, in turn, provided a sense of purpose and direction that enhanced hope and motivation:

> Consider the religious view of a forgiving, merciful, all-powerful God who is in control of life's circumstances and even the eternity that is beyond life, who is interested… and responds to…pleas. (Koenig and Larson 2001, pp. 71–2)

For anyone working with patients/clients as a chaplain or advocate in whatever service, hope can be a rare commodity and could often be maxi-

---

[6] MacIntyre (1985) says that there is 'at least one virtue recognised by the tradition which cannot be specified at all except with reference to the wholeness of human life—the virtue of integrity or constancy' (Hauerwas and Berkman 2005, p. 87) (see 4.2 (b) (v) and the advocacy quality of integrity).

mised. Spiritual assessment including 'hope' belongs to an area which is under consideration in terms of providing a model of care which combines a therapeutic purpose for staff, including chaplains, and possibly for advocates, but which above all should lead to outcomes for clients or patients. In one mental health trust, spiritual assessment training was given within the joint service-user and staff sessions through the 'Recovery College.' There are a number of models of spiritual assessment, and the 'HOPE tool' has been often described and has been used in work with mental health patients. I will now look at this further and how this relates to advocacy.

Raffay (2011) wrote that the best of the 'readily available assessment tools' is the HOPE tool (citing Anandarajah and Hight 2001), whose greatest strength lies in the ease with which it can be used on a busy assessment ward. The acronym HOPE, which can be remembered and used by a 'skilled clinician' in the natural course of an 'easy-flowing conversation,' stands for:

'H: sources of hope, meaning, comfort, strength, peace, love and connection
   O: organized religion
   P: personal spirituality and practices
   E: effects on medical care and end-of-life issues.'(Anandarajah and Hight 2001; Raffay 2011, p. 61)

The HOPE tool and other assessment methods have been discussed in the public arena (Eagger 2005a, b). There is further evidence of the successful use of the HOPE tool in recent work with mental health service-users: within the framework of an occupational therapy activity, users were asked questions about what gave their lives meaning, their experience of formal faith, about their personal use of practices and how the responses could affect their treatment. There is no reason why this tool, which seeks to bring spiritual and religious comfort and direction, could not be used by independent advocates to have a broad understanding of what a client's social, emotional and cultural needs are, including the spiritual, especially if the advocate is not familiar with the background of their client in a first-hand way. Two examples from the data are relevant: Sam spoke of Vietnamese cultural and religious expectations, and how discrimination and misunderstanding could lead to a wrong diagnosis; and Norah of how she wanted to familiarise herself with the Asian and Hindu (as well as Roman Catholic) background of a dual heritage client so that he could draw strength from his mixed religious roots. The cultural and religious hopes of advocacy clients informed the equality-based approaches of their advocates. According to Wilkinson and Pickett (2010), given the higher level of mental ill health in more unequal countries, of which the UK is one, the role of mental health assessment here in community and residential services, which includes 'spiritual assessment,' is vital.[7] Finally, St. Paul wrote that 'love… always hopes…' (1 Corinthians 13:6, Bible) and it is the action of the advocate (in the process described as Action Based on Equality), and on behalf of those clients with or without capacity to make their own decisions, to build a hopeful future based on equal spiritual rights and religious principles which individuals and faiths espouse.

I now move on to the third of the Pauline triad of virtues, 'charity' or 'love,' and reflect on compassion as an ingredient of care in the NHS and in pastoral activity such as chaplaincy.

3.5.3   Kindness and Compassion as Support and Love

In verse 11 of the famous 'Hymn to Love' in which St. Paul extols the cardinal virtue, his words are often translated as 'love endures all things' (1 Corinthians 13:11, Bible). According to Barrett (1971), this can also be construed as 'love supports all things,' through reference to the saying of Simeon the Just (3 BC) that the world is sustained by the Law, the Service (of the Jewish temple) and acts of kindness. With the sense of sustenance linked with the particular verbal usage in Greek, related to the word for 'roof,' one could render this as 'love is the support of the world' (Barrett 1971, p. 304). The term 'support' is also prevalent in the world of social care and advocacy, as in the 'support-worker' role. Wright (1992), in fact, discussed a 'hermeneutic of love' using the term 'sensitive critical realism'

---

[7] 'In Germany, Italy, Japan and Spain, fewer than 1 in 10 people had been mentally ill within the previous year; in Australia, Canada, New Zealand and the UK the numbers are more than 1 in 5 people; and in the USA… more than 1 in 4' (Wilkinson and Pickett 2010, p. 67).

to apply to the reading of texts (N. T. Wright 1992, pp. 63–4). The above connotations would seem to be sympathetic with the view of spirituality which Critical Realist Bhaskar advanced, for when asked for a definition of spirituality, he announced from his basis in Eastern religion:

> Spirituality is total, consummate love – adoration – for everything that exists and has value in its own right. A love which carries with it boundless energy and respect for all forms of being… through the power of our love – our creativity – we can change ourselves and change the world. (Bhaskar 2002b, p. 93)

The narrower Christian concept of charity or 'love' of St. Paul is a more personal and behaviourist depiction of spirituality—'It does not boast… is not easily angered… always protects' (1 Corinthians 13: 4–7, Bible). In his later work, Hauerwas (2005) suggested that virtues such as trust and love only make sense in context since all 'communities require a sense of hope in the future and… witness to the necessity of love for sustaining relationships.' These 'traditional theological virtues' of faith, hope and love also sustain the church, as they do any community. A focus on the universal value of Christian virtues is then underlain by reference to the second letter to the Corinthians, which in the literal Greek translation is emphatic since there is no definite article.

> 'If anyone is in Christ… *new creation*! The old has gone, the new has come!' (2 Corinthians 5:16–17, Bible)

With reference to the 'realisation' of God's kingdom both then and now, the community of a new age continues to exist in the old age but makes virtues central (Hauerwas and Berkman 2005, pp. 378–9). Compassion and love are theologically critical for Hauerwas, who referred to the Church as how a faithful community should be understood. Reverting to 1 Corinthians 13 (Bible), it is God alone who can love spontaneously and without motivation, and love is a direct expression of God (Nygren cited in Barrett 1971, p. 310). Human expressions of compassion, although prompted by the divine, are often defective, and can undermine the claims of the Church, or any spiritual (or professional) community, to be virtuously representative of the divine any more than any non-religious, moral entity. Thus the behaviour of a church community, called to be exemplary, could be about power-grabbing, rather than as a demonstration of 'Christ-like love.' Anthony of Sourozh wrote:

> It seems to me... that the Church must never speak from a position of strength. It ought not to be one of the forces influencing this or that State. The Church ought to be, if you will, just as powerless as God himself which does not coerce but which calls and unveils the beauty and the truth of things without imposing them. As soon as the Church begins to exercise power, it loses its most profound characteristic which is divine love – the understanding of those it is called to save and not to smash. (Metropolitan-Anthony-Bloom 2012).

This self-emptying, sacrificial love, Metropolitan Anthony seems to say, must have an impact on the institutional church, but this could apply also to health and social care institutions in which advocates and chaplains move. I was grateful to a service-user who shared the above quotation with me and for her views of its implications for effective public engagement.[8] From the nursing field, the notion of 'compassion' is a helpful elaboration. A virtue that the individual cultivates as part of his or her character, it redefines love as 'strengthening... virtuous intention and practices and a deepening of the disposition to do the morally right thing even when no one is watching.' For Bradshaw (2009) there should be 'congruence' between the interior and exterior dimensions of moral acts, and compassion is love acted out in practice (Bradshaw 2009, p. 466).

The theological meaning of Christian love, *agape* (Gr.), is thus contained in both of my emergent guiding principles, namely Reconstructed Empowerment and Action Based on Equality, as they were elicited as analytical categories. These principles also carry what I have considered here as Christian notions of disempowerment and re-empowerment and equalisation, but aspects of these are seen in other spiritual traditions and texts. They are most essentially evoked in the practical outworking

---

[8] She commented: *'My feeling is this [Anthony of Sourozh quotation] beautifully expresses what we are trying to achieve in terms of redressing the balance of power between any seemingly omnipotent organization, such as a certain very wealthy Borough which shall remain nameless, or indeed any public body that resists the shift in power that effective public engagement represents'* (Personal communication 2012).

of one's love for the divine in monotheistic faiths, in the injunction to love the (Hebrew) Yahweh and to love (or empower) one's neighbour as oneself (see Deuteronomy 6:4–9; Mark 12:29–30, Bible). Love expressed in care (in nursing) was seen as the 'normative moral practice of compassionate help' for the stranger in need in terms of being one's brother's keeper (Bradshaw 2009, pp. 465–6). The practice of 'equalising' in almsgiving (Zakat) in Islam (see Sura 2:40, Koran) and the concrete action of compassion in the parable of the Good Samaritan (Luke 10:25–37, Bible) also bear this out, most of which have been alluded to above (1.2).

In this chapter so far I have begun to correlate the spiritual or theological uses of advocacy, how chaplains may benefit from advocacy, with the advantages which advocates may draw from spiritual and theological practices. Theological aspects of love and compassion will be referenced further below as a constituent element in the recovery of a traditional nursing model, which Bradshaw (2004) advocated. I referred above to advocacy as offering spiritual hospitality. It is in this context that I want to consider what kind of spiritual support or training will sustain advocates in the service which they are called to provide (Hauerwas and Berkman 2005, pp. 554, 548). This could have consequences for equality required both by the Human Rights Act and by religious principles, namely the injunction to love one's neighbour, and the Golden Rule (e.g. 'Do as you would be done by' and Matthew 7:1, Bible). From these elements it was accordingly possible to think about spiritual as well as religious rights, and how they link, along with health and social care rights, to the Disability Discrimination Act 2007, the Equalities Act 2010, the Mental Health and Mental Capacity Acts as well as to the Human Rights Act, the Care Act 2014 (see 1.6) and to some of the aspects which are current in the well-being debate rehearsed above. Any training would need to be housed within this human equalities framework but extended to include spiritual and cultural elements. The triple virtues of St. Paul have provided a practical theological route for this to take place, as I have shown.

In the next section I propose that independent advocacy requires some kind of joint training initiative or resource base within the practice whereby equal spiritual rights may be protected and developed. For that to take place a tradition and expectation of spiritual struggle is needed, parallel and related to that found in religion and theology.

4   How 'Spirituality Advocates' and Nursing Theory Assist Towards a Practical Theology of Advocacy

4.1   Chaplaincy Develops Spirituality Advocates

Within at least two Mental Health NHS trusts in England, the concepts of spirituality and advocacy have been combined in the role which has become known as the 'spirituality advocate' or, elsewhere, 'champion'. The chaplain Richard Harlow developed the idea in order to raise the level of awareness of nursing staff about the place of spirituality and faith within their role in assessment of the patient. A spirituality advocate was not a job in itself but a role which a particular healthcare professional on a ward (probably a nurse or possibly an occupational therapist) would offer, or be asked to assume, within an existing paid post. It was Harlow (2010) therefore who described how spiritual assessment would work in relation to safeguarding, and by maintaining trust standards as part of developing a 'Spiritual Strategy' for a trust:

> The role of the spirituality advocate is to champion the inclusion of the spiritual domain in the holistic care of service users and their carers, to improve the care… and to embed service improvements in the religion and belief domain of the Single Equality Scheme. (Harlow 2010)

Advocates were to 'model individual good practice,' argued Harlow, because their 'chief function is to assist the multi-disciplinary team' in recognising and responding to the spiritual and religious needs of service-users and carers within a 'recovery framework' (Harlow 2010, p. 620). Harlow's work commended itself to other chaplaincy trusts via the chaplaincy network, and, influenced by Harlow, another chaplaincy team then produced a similar policy and a training package from its Department of Spiritual and Pastoral Care. At the time these were activities which this 'adopter' spiritual care department saw as important for spirituality advocacy: 'spiritual care assessment as part of the recovery process, different approaches to mapping spirituality and identity, work with faith and spiritual communities, blocks to responding to the spiritual dimension, spirituality and mental health care' (G. Harrison 2011).

The actual job description of a spirituality advocate was set out by the originating trust as firstly being able to use the 'spiritual assessment tool,' which was based on the HOPE questionnaire. This was referred to above (6.3.5.), typified here as Reconstructing Empowerment in action. The job description also involved acting as a resource for information— for example, chaplaincy leaflets/posters/religious festival calendars—then keeping oversight of any sacred space (or chapel) on the unit (i.e. individual ward) to ensure it is a safe and welcoming space. A spirituality advocate would act as a link with chaplains (assuming that there was a chaplaincy available) and enhance a referral system. Johnson and Harlow (2011) explained what a 'spiritual advocate' would do, namely, challenge stigma or discrimination—which related to the anti-stigma role of advocates in this study using Action Based on Equality—and attend initial and ongoing training for advocates, and in this role would also build knowledge of spirituality and religion and the understanding of the role itself (S. Johnson and Harlow 2011).

Harlow (2010) continued by describing the nature of his understanding of 'Spirituality Advocates.' They need to be 'flexible in their thinking' about religious and belief diversity, be willing to learn and have an awareness of personal beliefs and mindsets around spirituality; they also need to be willing to tackle embedded stigma or prejudice and be able to communicate effectively. However, they would also be trained for the specific requirements of the role (Harlow 2010, p. 620). It remains to be seen whether this role would be a contractual requirement or a voluntary role. Nevertheless, a 'spirituality broker' is necessary in a climate where, for example, mental health NHS trusts are not employing chaplains but relying on volunteers. Risks may exist in that those selected to be champions do not fully understand the range and detailed varied expressions of religious belief which may be around in a busy London trust, but clear benefits would be drawn from individuals in nursing roles who were themselves rooted in religious traditions, so that they appropriately develop their understanding of St. Paul's teaching on love officially within the health service.

A possible greater level of cooperation between mental health chaplaincy and advocacy practitioners was signalled in that spiritual care professionals were using the term 'advocate' within their strategic aims and that their duties included 'responding to the spiritual and religious needs of service users' (Harlow 2010, p. 620). It was true that independent advocates needed to consider spiritual needs amongst a whole range of other needs which a client may need supporting with. The spirituality advocate focused on the spiritual needs; the 'secular' independent advocate will include social, spiritual and cultural needs in her action. In the final section of this chapter, I will make the link between theological virtue, spirituality and advocacy, and between spirituality and nursing, an area in which relatively more systematic work has been done.

4.2   Lessons from Nursing Theory for a Virtuous Spirituality of Advocacy

I explained why I chose chaplaincy as a comparator profession in order to scrutinise advocacy 'faithfully' within the discipline of Practical Theology. It was not that other fields were not considering spirituality and theology in some depth which would be pertinent to advocacy, and therefore I alluded to youth ministry and spiritual accompaniment as well as nursing. For these reasons—and within the explanation-building case study method which I use—I will bring input from this related practice area and triangulate further in this creative conversation about advocacy, with the positioning of one aspect of nursing.

Bradshaw's (1994) argument for the rehabilitation of a classical covenant-based 'Lamp tradition' and an explicitly Christian model of nursing care was set up as a riposte to what she viewed as the ways that the theories of Florence Nightingale and Cicely Saunders— the founder of the hospice movement—had been supplanted. Bradshaw (1994), cited in McSherry and Ross (2010), found that spiritual, and specifically Christian, love to be ideally central to nursing practice. Although the practice of advocacy was generally located in a secular paradigm and it defined itself against nursing or social work, this study has parallel intentions to Bradshaw's. The extract below captures the tenor of her argument:

The spiritual dimension of nursing in the covenant meta-paradigm is the meaning of nursing itself. It is the definition of care now being so desperately sought by nursing writers... the undermining of the Judeo-Christian foundations of nursing care has resulted in a problem of defining the concept of care itself. It is interesting that Griffin (1983), for example, who tries unsatisfactorily to delineate the components of care from philosophy, finally concludes: 'perhaps, it might not be altogether too far-fetched to identify a dominant emotion in caring as a kind of love' (Griffin 1983, p. 294). The power of the classical tradition is precisely here, at this point of uncertainty, because it defines this kind of love theologically as rooted in the covenant. Love is not merely, as Griffin suggests, a 'dominant emotion' dependent on the capriciousness of the nurse's human nature, but a covenant gift of agape which springs from creation, from the source of love and the meaning of care. (Ann Bradshaw 1994, p. 330)

Bradshaw's focus on the provenance of love helps to place the teaching of Wolfensberger, cited above, in the context of a Practical Theology of advocacy. Of further relevance to the theme of this study was Bradshaw's link between the theological concept of the 'advocate,' which I discussed above, and specific nursing care. The New Testament theologian Brown (1971) contributed with the...

Greek word for the Holy Spirit, Paraclete, which is variously translated as 'advocate', 'comforter', 'guide', 'he who comes alongside', 'teacher', and 'he who bears witness' (R. E. Brown 1971, pp. 1135–1137). This expresses the nature of God, his love as agape, and it is a description of the nurse's role. Agape, as the gift of the Holy Spirit, is the fulfilment of nursing and the meaning of spiritual care... as Barth has shown, *agape*, compassion, fellow-feeling, is precisely love that is not moderated, that is unconditional and that demands that the carer offers an unselfish devotion. (Ann Bradshaw 1994, p. 322)

While Bradshaw's study had its weaknesses—in failing to take account of the impact of nursing professionalisation on practice—the call for a re-evaluation of the importance of classical spiritual concepts in relation to this particular vocation was a dimension I wanted to explore in interviews with my participants as they spoke about their experience or perceptions of advocacy, an emergent independent and holistic tradition and practice. Using understandings from theology and philosophy, therefore, and with reference to virtue ethics and critical realism approaches, I have constructed a model for advocacy. This model encompasses and draws attention to spiritual and theological concerns, with Reconstructed Empowerment and Action Based on Equality as centripetal forces within it. But it does not ignore awareness of the distinctive history and practice of advocacy located in the interstices of the secular expression of health and social care in the UK, and which are marked by a sense of professionalisation in the making.

Although the independent advocates and clients interviewed rarely made an explicit connection between advocacy and spirituality or religion, as the author I have noted implicit comparisons and contrasts between the two areas in the combination of interviews with advocates and spiritual care coordinators. Sam said that an *'equaliser'* must try to support clients to have access to *'their rights as though they didn't have a disability or whatever it is that defines the client group'* (see Sam 2008, February 13). The notion that the advocacy role consisted in ensuring equality was raised by participants Nebi and Sam from different sources. The principle point of partnership and the need to conduct a levelling exercise, as Sam described, were sharply expressed by both participants. In terms of his advocating for individuals from a religious and pastoral perspective, the chaplain Norman's views resonated with the above:

> *I don't know how secular advocates would define their role but I would define it as one of solidarity, one of empowerment, one of levelling out the imbalances of power...* (Norman and Colin 2008, September 11)

These views were made explicit in the narrative and linked to principles of charitable behaviour in Judaeo-Christian and in Islamic theology. For example, the foundational injunction of the Torah, the Shema, to love Yahweh and one's neighbour as oneself (Deuteronomy 6:4–9; Mark 12:29–30, Bible); the practice of alms-giving (Zakat) in Islam; and the practical action of compassion exemplified in Christ's teaching in the parable of the Good Samaritan (Luke 10:25–37, Bible) were related, through examples and from interviews, to the practice of advocacy. Although such a comparison may be anathema to some advocates and secularists, it may be acceptable when framed in terms of 'well-being,' which was also reflected earlier in the book (see above, 2.1.6. and 6.1.3.).

Layard (2009) was a proponent of well-being, and this also became a concept which was concretised in statutory measures in the UK from 2010 through the introduction of Health and Well-Being Boards and various political discourses developments. The Health and Social Care Act 2012/2014 has set in place these boards, which have responsibility for PPI through 'Healthwatch,' a re-incarnation of what was previously known as LINkS (Anonymous 2011). Layard may not hold theological views, but nonetheless noted the need for altruistic direction:

We desperately need a social norm in which the good of others figures more prominently in our personal goals. (Layard 2009, September 14)

4.3   Reconstructed Empowerment, Action Based on Equality, Spiritual Assessment and IMCA Reporting

The twin concepts of Reconstructed Empowerment and Action Based on Equality represented the addition of a holistic, spiritual and theological approach to independent advocacy. This synthesis of findings formed an interpretation which could be developed in a training programme which includes reference to the spirituality of nursing, the 'use of self' (5.4(d)) or spiritual assessment, in order conceivably to establish a stronger basis for advocacy theory and practice. IMCA practitioners provide a practical role and a specific form of advocacy within England and Wales today. I showed this earlier, and also provided case studies elsewhere of how advocacy helped clients with ABI using aspects of spiritual assessment (see Chap. 2 and Morgan 2011a). IMCA guidance stated that 'it is not possible for IMCAs to be able to know everything about a person when it comes to their beliefs or values.' It noted the importance of attempting to find out how their values (which is also true for wishes and prefer-ences) can impact on a decision. For example, 'if a person was born into a particular faith, do they still practise this?' If not, is this a choice or determined by circumstances—for example, if they have been unable to leave the house for some time and have therefore been unable to attend a place of worship? Alternatively, according to the guidance, if they have or had non-religious, cultural or lifestyle-related beliefs and attitudes that have been an integral aspect of their identity, it would be important to investigate these in order to determine their relevance to the decision and ways in which they may be promoted or upheld for the client (Action-for-Advocacy 2011, pp. 34–5).

In the light of the above, I suggested in the specific example of ABI, that it may be helpful for all healthcare professionals including IMCAs (and any working or caring for vulnerable people) to learn from the tools of spiritual assessment, tools which are being used increasingly by nursing staff and chaplains/spiritual care coordinators in mental health trusts and some staff in acute hospitals (see Eagger 2005a; Morgan 2011a, pp. 214–5).

A final example from a textbook on the subject of law and safeguarding vulnerable adults pinpointed the IMCA's role as one that 'cannot be underestimated... [having]

> the scope to have enormous influence for individuals who are unable to state clearly what they want, and are assessed to be unable to make certain decisions. This client group represents some of most vulnerable and potentially disempowered people in society.' (Pritchard 2009, p. 151)

Pritchard continued to note how overlooked and marginalised such clients may be: older people with dementia and no family remaining, a young retired person with a brain injury with no known contacts, a younger person with a learning disability whose parents are no longer able to take decisions for her. For these and other people, the resources of advocacy exist and are provided through commissioning arrangements by the state. This would not have been so were it not for a history and the recent activity of advocacy organisations, which, as I showed, had (sometimes subtle) spiritual or theological ramifications of which cognizance can usefully be taken. Christian theology typically and historically characterised such activity, albeit in health and social care, as 'pure religion' in supporting 'widows' and 'orphans' (James 1:27, Bible). As voluntary organisations and their diverse workforce seek to meet advocacy needs, a broader disciplinary, theoretical and skills base is required for advocacy practice. The need for this has been demonstrated in this book. Such a skill-set will include not only practical knowledge and application but the capacity to think, problem-solve, reflect holistically and spiritually, and to draw on established and appropriate theological resources. Indeed the case study above ('use of self') gave an example of a practice which could provide a framework for advocates and chaplains to mutually re-structure their working models in the context of this creative theological conversation.

5   Conclusion

In this chapter I amplified voices from earlier sections of the narrative, such as the literature and conversational sections, and used the themes of Reconstructed Empowerment and Action Based on Equality to achieve this, within the discipline of Practical Theology with reference to Professional Studies. This work is intended to make up a deficit in spiritual discourse in health and social care (and argue for its prima facie purpose) and specifically to establish links between theology, spirituality and advocacy practice. The purpose, as stated, will to be to add to the debate about the professionalisation of advocacy by interrogating the practice within the discipline of practical theology, in short, to think faithfully (through eyes which respect spirituality and faith values) about advocacy. As explained in previous chapters, the aim of the book is to make connections, within independent voluntary organisations, between advocacy and PPI and personal, theological and spiritual development, and to raise the volume of voices which speak meaning into these topics.

The key questions and theories from virtue ethics were vehicles which I used to link advocacy with chaplaincy and spirituality in mental health, and the approach to practice called spiritual assessment. In Sect. 1 wanted to engineer a spiritual convergence using the integrative model of hospitality with the often conceived secular and rights-based identity of independent advocacy. In Sect. 2 I looked at definitions of spiritual 'well-being' in the light of Aristotle and a new application of virtue ethics. Then in the process of Sect. 3 I considered the spiritual and theological impact of virtue ethics on the practice of advocacy, moved through 'spiritual rights' and social developments, consolidated this position as 'Deep Advocacy' and re-interpreted the analytical perspectives, Reconstructed Empowerment and Action based on Equality, based on a reading of St. Paul in 1 Corinthians 13 (Bible). Finally in Sect. 4 I built on this to suggest a theological interpretation of advocacy practice, which led to possible courses of action for further development. I drew attention again to the discipline of nursing which has been, and is, a crucial arena for the exploration and application of spiritual assessment in its own right. This was justified, therefore, as a prism through which to consider comparisons between the reaches which advocacy and chaplaincy respectively demonstrate, combined in a new development of the 'spirituality advocate' or champion. Discussion of spiritualities of nursing, chaplaincy and advocacy routed the conversation from the model of virtue ethics back to a deepened theory of advocacy practice in which I referenced the voices of participants and, for example, Wolfensberger. I juxtaposed the innovation of 'spirituality advocates' with another voice from nursing, a field from which we heard intermittently throughout the narrative, to suggest a theological definition and to shed light on one technical aspect of advocacy, IMCA reporting practice (McSherry et al. 2008; McSherry and Jamieson 2011; McSherry and Ross 2010).

The fusion shows the importance that I attributed to the professional role of independent advocates, illustrated with reference to the case studies where the most vulnerable client could be supported or signposted in a spiritually or theologically competent way by an IMCA practitioner, using tools of spiritual assessment.

7

Spirit of Advocacy

1   Summary of Argument

The argument of this book is related to issues around the development of advocacy as a professionalised occupation in England and Wales from 2005 onwards. As the statutory requirement for IMCAs and IMHAs passed into English and Welsh law in 2007 and 2009, respectively, I showed how this highlighted the growing significance of advocacy in health and social care and the emergence of these particular roles as occupations undergoing professionalisation. Social policy changes, the advancing consciousness of human rights and broader awareness of cultural and spiritual influences occurring in the same areas evidenced the above.

These social and cultural pressures were shown to have affected the evolution of advocacy as an occupation as it was shaped into a profession. Independent advocacy has its roots in altruistic and spiritual soil, and specifically in its Western European and, to some extent, American expressions, within the field of theology. Wolfensberger drew on more contemporary Scandinavian versions, which he imported into the US

© The Author(s) 2017   **225**
G. Morgan, *Independent Advocacy and Spiritual Care*,
DOI 10.1057/978-1-137-53125-4_7

and which then arrived in other parts of Europe. In the scope of literature, therefore, advocacy was discerned in early civil, political and human rights movements, mental health history and nursing philosophy; there was also continuity with the voices which heralded the arrival of self-conscious advocacy in the twentieth and twenty-first centuries. The increase in the literature of spirituality and mental health, concepts of well-being, empowerment and democratisation in the rising service-user movement were tidal events which pointed to a spirituality of advocacy.

The role of an advocate, as an independent agent or witness, was distinct from the role which a paid employee of a trust or local authority, such as a nurse or a social worker, could play. Furthermore, the extension of these roles (nurse, social worker) to cover what an independent 'advocate' would, or could, do was rejected. Consequently this led to an independent 'caring' gap needing to be filled, one which voluntary sector organisations, funded increasingly by central government, could fill. Thus advocacy came to be separated from 'the system' in order to be better able to support and represent clients, patients or service-users, but in the process it also acquired, in its new-found professionalisation, specific training needs. With the coming of age of advocacy, the question arose of whether there is a theoretical paucity in view of what legislative statutes, or social workers, consultants or psychiatrists now expect of advocates. Also, because of its spiritual history, approaching advocacy in the framework of Practical Theology enhanced its theological basis and refreshed its ethical components.

For the above reasons in Chaps. 4 and 5 (and using a case study method) I turned to the voluntary and community organisations where I worked in the advocacy sector from 2005 to 2011. Observations of the identity of the advocate via the experiences of a number of selected advocacy practitioners and those of their clients revealed new facts which combine to improve aspects of advocacy practice. The voices of advocates, self-advocates and clients defined normatively the essence of advocacy practice and experience. In addition, conversations were constructed with voices from another profession, namely, chaplains, and, to a limited extent, from nursing, from within the discipline of Practical Theology, and these were arbitrated by analytical models which apply spiritually and theologically constructed models of empowerment or equal rights—Reconstructed Empowerment and Action Based on Equality. Based on the information, these mapped, respectively, the delicate approach advocates adopt to support clients with diminished or no capacity for certain decisions and the actions which are taken by them in relation to clients to rebalance their equality legally and spiritually. These themes were interwoven in the text and are expanded in the synthesis of Chap. 6. Multiple sources also lent increased validity and reliability to the argument.

The inclusion of chaplains alongside advocates aided deeper excavation into the foundations and implications of independent advocacy from a spiritual and Christian point of view, within the implied limits of that scheme. Parallel to independent advocacy, healthcare chaplaincy is a role which exists to support patients, their relatives and staff but only (up to most recent times) on the territory of healthcare trusts in the NHS in England and Wales. Whilst statutory independent advocacy has professional boundaries, there are positive ambiguities with 'voluntary' citizen advocacy, which were mined. Alongside this, existing from the birth of the NHS in 1948, spiritual care exercised in the chaplaincy service in the NHS is a religious and ministerial function which connects with historical faith communities and has a similar semi-independent role in relation to the National Health Service. The fact that this will take place within the format of the discipline of Practical Theology gave theological force to my findings.

The history of professionalisation, with which I am concerned in advocacy, bears similarities with that of chaplaincy. Therefore the merger of insights from secular and faith-based advocates, the latter being those who are mostly, but not exclusively, employed as chaplains, took place to form a particular independent perspective. Independence is important for advocates and, whilst there is an element of independence in chaplaincy, it is inevitable that chaplains will be employed by NHS trusts and cannot therefore be seen as advocates in the way that advocacy organisations would define the role. The independence of advocates could be compromised by the fact that being statutory from 2007 brought increasingly boundaried behaviours to which the traditional 'citizen advocate' (mentioned above) was resistant, the sum of which contributed to a profoundly spiritual stance in the ongoing conversation.

It is independence within professional advocacy which gives meaning to the activity. Advocacy is commonly understood as a statutory human rights-based expression, much of which is strongly established in UK advocacy legislation. I argued that these policies locate a *conduit* for principles of culture and faith to apply to independent advocacy, underlining why the field of Practical Theology was the best in which to achieve this. How NHS-funded chaplaincy works was not the subject of this book, but similarities with advocacy came from the shared quasi-independent perspective, and it was the basis on which I chose to bring in chaplaincy as a comparator profession, or conversational partner. Despite its shorter history, I found that advocacy was in some ways more secure and durable as a profession than chaplaincy, on account of its human rights and secular basis, and with its comparatively greater level of acceptability due to a gain in status in the last 20 years. The argument focused on advocacy on account of its similar support role to chaplaincy, and where the advocate, like the chaplain, could not ever be a decision-maker. Advocacy thus contributed to an understanding of the role of chaplaincy and should have similar benefits for other faith-based organisations in the community. This material relates to the second and third key questions: Qs 2 and 3.

The expansion of literature in spirituality and mental health was something which all chaplains or spiritual care coordinators should be aware of, and it represented (especially with emphases on spiritual assessment) another important angle for the advocacy sector to take account of. Together this suggested that both mental health chaplaincy and spirituality, and mental health theory and some aspects of nursing, which I set out in relation to the literature, were dimensions which benefit from a link with professional advocacy. This connection was broadened and deepened by the exploration of the information from my interview participants.

Against the background of a portrait of the professional activity and reflexivity in the area studied, a culturally and spiritually appropriate model of advocacy based in the discipline of Practical Theology was outlined. Although advocacy at first appeared to be a thoroughly secular occupation, which fulfils a basic humanistic signposting role, voices from advocacy, chaplaincy, nursing philosophy, the relevant literature and public policy were critically correlated to present a theologically informed, virtue ethics-related approach to independent advocacy. Having listened to the voices from all groups, the synthesising practice models of Reconstructed Empowerment and Action Based on Equality were emblematic of this. The uses (or abuses) of power and equal (or unequal) rights are the substance of advocacy, and these 'new' models integrated religious or spiritual elements into advocacy practice within the established remit of Practical Theology. Spiritual, theological or 'faithful' capital is, I argued, every individual's human right, is at the heart of independent advocacy and has implications for the way religious, Christian (for example), and everyday communities form themselves; this resulted in the description 'spiritual rights.' The concepts of Reconstructed Empowerment and Action Based on Equality were related to the third key question, in a new quasi-therapeutic, although enduringly independent and appropriately culturally and spiritually sensitive, space. As well as what spirituality and chaplaincy can bring to advocacy, the question of what independent advocacy may have to say to chaplaincy was raised within the creative and critical conversation. This was why so much attention was given to the voices of participants.

2   Recommendations for Practice

As indicated, independent advocacy happens in a variety of modes (instructed and non-instructed, non-statutory and statutory) and in a diversity of schemes, some focused on particular client groups or other (elderly, BAME, and so on). It also has distinctive dimensions in UK social policy and in safeguarding the vulnerable, including children. With its peculiar history as a social movement and contested emergent status as a service, advocacy has not always conversed constructively with other professions. In this book I have documented an account of advocacy and provided an engagement between advocacy and statutory spiritual and pastoral care (or chaplaincy) in order to understand what both disciplines could learn from one another. Although both seem to be marginal to health and social care, political, economic and community developments in the UK—the time of austerity and swinge-ing benefit cuts for the disabled—make independent advocacy more needful than ever. Recommendations which emerged from the study were as follows.

2.1   Training for Paid and Volunteer Advocates

Culture and spirituality are important factors for non-statutory and statutory independent advocates to bear in mind in their support for individuals, and, even though statutory advocacy training is understandably outcome- and decision-oriented, greater attention should be given to standard citizen advocate approaches to individuals, including the history of advocacy, which view them holistically. This could be reflected in more specific culture, religion, or spirituality-based training for full-time and volunteer advocates within advocacy schemes, and in the current Department of Health training requirements for IMCAs and IMHAs, who need to consider clients' best interests. The strengths of volunteer and learning disability advocacy have been made clear in relation to the history of the movement. With increasing reliance on volunteers in the sharper financial climate, schemes themselves will need to consider how their paid statutory and volunteer advocates use their own transferable skills within training and relate with other professional domains, for example, Occupational Therapy or chaplaincy, for the benefit of clients. Cooperation between advocacy training initiatives and spiritual and pastoral care departments would be important in agreeing what could be achieved; a practical outcome could be a common training module.

2.2   Reflective Practice with Spiritual Care

For practitioner advocates the supervision and ability to reflect on their practice will often depend on the management in the advocacy scheme which employs them or to which they are responsible as volunteers. For statutory advocates, in particular IMCAs, the output of reports for decision-makers in social care and the NHS, will be the criteria against which, with the help of their supervisors in regular monthly meetings, they are able to reflect critically upon their practice. In chaplaincy, although reports are not an expectation, the clinical supervision process, which is best practice although not obligatory, may generate a more therapeutic and philosophical reflectivity. In fact, it should also feed back into the personal and professional practice and well-being of the minister of religion of whatever hue and help her to innovate in practical and public theology. I have shown that the personal ownership of one's professional development and responsibility for improving practice, which ideally exists in spiritual and pastoral care, could be usefully transferred to advocacy by considering features such as, for example, virtue ethics and theology, the 'use of self,' or spiritual assessment. This will increase authenticity and credibility within the emergent field of statutory independent advocacy practice and have implications for advocacy more broadly.

2.3   Advocacy Management

Within statutory independent advocacy (IMCA), raw data about IMCA referrals across England are sent in to the Department of Health national database maintained by the Health and Social Care Information Centre. This leads to the generation of an Annual Report, which in 2011–2012 showed that referrals had increased by 9 % over the previous year ((DoH) 2013). Some reflective material from advocates was included in this report which generally related to the quality of the outcomes. IMCA advocacy is an untypical form of advocacy in that it is centrally managed and focused on the most vulnerable individuals clearly identified by the system. Disciplined management techniques driven by the bureaucracy of the Department of Health could helpfully be used to draw out even more qualitative material from the IMCA advocates, as well as other advocates, as part of their supervision (set out in training requirements) and their own professional development. The character of the qualitative data could be led by the research questions used and be reflected upon using approaches captured in my interview accounts. Conceptual categories such as Reconstructed Empowerment and Action Based on Equality or Deep Advocacy can provide pointers for this. This process could embed practice and guard against attrition within some schemes.

2.4   Advocacy in Society

I have placed independent advocacy in a particular social and political context and suggested that statutory advocacy and the limited provision of non-statutory advocacy means that many more people could benefit from the service than currently do so, especially the most vulnerable, whose exposed position is often reported in media. There is a need for voluntary and religious organisations to join together and consider ways of providing 'one-stop advocacy.' Arguably these kind of services already exist without dignifying the activity as 'advocacy,' but the voluntary sector, which generally hosts advocacy initiatives, could be funded to be more pro-active with other community and spiritual organisations in order to extend a hand to known hard-to-reach groups and communities. This belongs with my call for a deeper, more spiritually integrated profession of advocacy.

3   What the Future May Hold

The interaction with spirituality and the use of the discipline of Practical Theology to set up a creative, critical conversation between the profession of advocacy and that of chaplaincy has led to a few areas for further investigation.

3.1   Further Conversations Between Advocacy and Chaplaincy

I have used some observed models of chaplaincy to scrutinise the development and practice of advocacy, which is very much an under-researched field; more research has comparably taken place in the field of chaplaincy studies. The theological dimension of this book makes it possible for chaplains or theologians to consider how principles of advocacy may be further related to various practical aspects of spiritual and pastoral care, or theology. How, for example, can a chaplain advocate independently for a patient who feels he is mistreated within an NHS trust when s/he is employed by that trust?

3.2   Conversations Between other Professional Fields and Advocacy

I have made reference to the growing literature linking spirituality with nursing. This would be a fruitful area for more thorough research in relation to advocacy. I alluded to the relationships which advocates have around their clients with other professionals, such as psychiatrists, social workers or occupational therapists. More structured thinking should be done in relation to models of practice and spirituality in these fields, and what impact such an interface could have on Practical Theology as well as on advocacy.

3.3   Advocacy, Well-Being Theory and Spirituality Studies

Well-being theory is a developing area of research, especially with the ascendancy of such terms within the social and political settlement in England with the Health and Social Care Acts 2012 and 2014 and the embedding of CCGs from April 2013. Individual and collective well-being often relates to culture, religion and spirituality; this is an area of research which has been highlighted as needing to progress. Insights from advocacy theory and practice and its correlation with spiritual care could be usefully applied to thinking about in what a flourishing life would consist. Similarly, advocacy could be related to the growing field of Spirituality Studies. This book has been framed in a mainly Christian context using Practical Theology. The context of Spirituality Studies would be a useful frame of reference to consider further cultural, ethnic or religious synergies which should be taken account of by all involved in advocacy.

4   Finale

The assumption of the overall study was that there was a deficit in terms of the capacity of the current practice of independent advocates to reflect upon their role, to be clear in their approach, and to gather as usefully as possible from existing theory and history in order to assemble a structural base for future development. That is not to say that a liberal, secular approach to advocacy has been ineffective thus far; on the contrary, without the impact of organisations such as the UKAN and the wonderful former A4A and the hundreds of national and local advocacy schemes (e.g. Rethink, Mind) that existed and reproduced themselves while being centred on the needs of their clients, independent advocacy would not be so centrally placed in the health and social care scene in the UK. I argued nevertheless that principles of Action Based on Equality and Reconstructed Empowerment induced from my evidence and imbued wisth a holistic or theological tone assisted in consolidating advocacy theory. Thus it could absorb a broader and richer philosophical, or even spiritual, diet, insofar as the discipline it was mixed with in these chapters was Practical Theology. Indeed, I have shown that the constituent elements in some histories of independent advocacy revealed 'faithful,' spiritual and often, but not exclusively, Christian theological depths which could be owned in further developments. In particular, one could consider the public-facing and statutory tasks which advocacy has to deal with, especially touching those who are without capacity to make certain decisions, or are vulnerable due to an impairment of mind.

Finally, in relation to whether independent advocacy or spiritual care initiatives could in themselves meet the needs of those who are 'unbefriended,' or desperately need support in a period of economic austerity, it is doubtful. But a society which upholds tangible safeguards, including expressions of independent advocacy flowing from the Mental Health and Mental Capacity Acts and the most recent ramifications of the Care Act 2014, redounds to the public good and is, I argue, more socially integrated. And alongside similar services, such as funded chaplaincy, which view the individual not only holistically but also in spiritual terms, together all must find new, efficient and practical ways to keep faith with the most vulnerable individuals and groups in that society, breathing forth life in the spirit of advocacy.

Appendix 1

Key Questions:

Q1. How does professionalisation affect the practice and experience of independent advocates?

Q2. How can the practice of advocacy be explained within the framework of the experience of advocacy practitioners, clients and spiritual care professionals or chaplains?

Q3. What philosophical or theological models (e.g. Christian ethics, virtue ethics) can be used to consider, better understand and move towards responses to questions Q1 and Q2?

Supplemental Key Questions:

SQ1. What are the strengths of unpaid roles as occupations, e.g. citizen or peer advocates, or chaplaincy volunteers?

SQ2. How is professionalisation affected by debates within schemes about the nature of advocacy practice?

SQ3. Is statutory advocacy in the UK necessary, or a waste of public money?

© The Author(s) 2017
G. Morgan, *Independent Advocacy and Spiritual Care*,
DOI 10.1057/978-1-137-53125-4

SQ4. Self-advocacy is a social movement. Statutory advocacy is a social service. Is this an irreconcilable paradox?

SQ5. Redress and complaints systems abound in the UK NHS and social care systems so why do we need independent advocates?

Appendix 2

List of participants – all personal names and organisation names have been changed

NB Most participants chose their own pseudonyms including all the advocacy clients

Beginning as a volunteer advocate while *Angela* was still working for her company for five years, the experience of supporting a friend was also formative for Angela as she advanced in responsibility in advocacy organisations using a trajectory which she had in common with other advocates.

Barry was a member of ISAP (Islingham Self Advocacy Project), a user group based in a college, for people with mild to moderate learning disabilities—and has himself had a citizen (volunteer) advocate for two years and has had issues with employment and in relation to caring for his wife with disabilities. Advocacy has supported him in this engagement.

Bella had been a volunteer citizen advocate for many years. Both Bella's and Norah's testimonies are valuable because they go back to the origin of this movement.

Bernard was a spiritual care coordinator in a number of hospitals/ Primary Care Trusts (PCTs) a priest with many years experience.

© The Author(s) 2017   **237**
G. Morgan, *Independent Advocacy and Spiritual Care*,
DOI 10.1057/978-1-137-53125-4

Colin was a chaplain in a hospital trust in a part-time capacity since he spent the rest of the time in the community.

Dorothy had been spiritual care coordinator for 20 years working in a psychiatric hospital.

Einstein, another member of ISAP, was a quiet individual. He did not say much but had become more confident with people he knew and had improved his communication through involvement with advocacy.

Fauzia was an advocate working with people with mental health problems both in hospitals and in the community.

Germaine was a key member of the HEARTH (Help Advocacy Reach Town Heath) group—a group of people with mild to moderate learning disabilities who are supported in self-advocacy to make choices within the borough—and is involved in the borough Partnership Board.

Beginning in an administrative role, *Jana* then progressed on to work in hospitals providing advocacy and servicing a patient's council, a form of group advocacy.

Janine had been involved in advocacy for only three years when I interviewed her. At first she started working with patients in hospitals, and then her organisation expanded and she worked in the community as well.

Karim was a Muslim spiritual care coordinator in a hospital trust; he enjoyed working with people of all faiths.

Kevin has been involved in 'getting people more choice and control' through his working life. He began by supporting volunteers, worked as a 'case manager,' support broker and then in advocacy management. Kevin mentioned that his inspiration was a family member who has learning disabilities who seeks 'to have a life that she wants to live.'

Louise was another member of HEARTH. Louise was involved in advocacy from when she was at school and is now a leading member of a Partnership Board.

Madonna was an original member of ISAP. Since being in the group she had developed in confidence and progressed from being a volunteer to being a paid tutor.

Maria came to advocacy through involvement in a legal role in supporting people with mental health issues. She spoke about how she picked it up as she went along and had experience in another public-facing role as well.

Maria came to advocacy through involvement in a legal role in supporting people with mental health issues. She spoke about how she picked it up as she went along and had experience in another public-facing role as well.

Michael was a founder member of HEARTH. He became involved through his social worker and has over ten years of involvement and activity in the group, within the borough.

Micky was a member of ISAP. He was by nature an individualist but the view of his self-advocacy group leader, which he owned, was that being part of the group has enabled him to be understood and accepted and to be more community-minded.

For *Nebi* the way-in to the profession of advocacy was through having been an interpreter and translator. He has progressed with the same organisation to a management position.

Nigel was spiritual care coordinator with management responsibility in a hospital trust.

Norah was a professional advocate of long standing, a coordinator of citizen advocates, and a citizen advocate with an advocacy organisation.

Norma was a keen younger ISAP member, who described how her helping (advocacy) skills in relation to her mother were assisted through group membership.

Noreen, also a member of ISAP, was married and had been working in an administrative job for the last five years, in a post that was created for people with learning disabilities. Noreen was very deaf and since being part of ISAP she has been confident to say when she did not hear what was said.

Olive was a new employee as a self-advocacy support worker in the advocacy sector. She had come to it as an alternative to being promoted to a management position because she wanted a role where she would not be 'out of contact with service-users.'

Peter was an advocate with advanced skills and someone with much experience of working with people with learning disabilities.

Another member of HEARTH, Pixy was excited to be involved in Partnership Board activities in the borough.

Robert, a member of ISAP, was knowledgeable and vocal in relation to disability discrimination. It was very difficult for him and his girlfriend (now wife) to get married: Robert encountered opposition from his wife's mother.

For *Ruth*, her advocacy career began when she was working in the private sector; she developed an interest in mental health and was attracted to her first post because it did not require specific qualifications (such as social work or nursing training). However, her experience in voluntary work helped. Moving on into management she then joined other organisations providing community advocacy and supporting the development of community advocacy.

Sam began volunteering when a teenager and professes a lifelong interest in the marginalised and supporting them. She has worked in a number of advocacy organisations in a variety of advocacy roles.

Sarah was a spiritual care coordinator/chaplain in a mental health trust. She began working as a chaplaincy volunteer in a hospital before being employed as a chaplain.

Scoby was an enthusiastic member of ISAP. He used to live in an institutional 'old school' service for people with learning disabilities and has been living in a supported living setting for 5 years.

Whitney became involved in self-advocacy in HEARTH through her keyworker and was supported with a change of accommodation.

Yolanda, another member of ISAP, had been working full-time in a standard employment environment for 20 years. She travelled every day on her own.

Zablon was a spiritual care coordinator in a hospital trust and also involved in a local church.

References

Action-for-Advocacy. (2002). *The Advocacy Charter*. Retrieved February 9, 2008, from http://www.aqvx59.dsl.pipex.com/Advocacy%20Charter2004.pdf

Action-for-Advocacy. (2006a). *A code of practice for Advocacy*. From http://www.aqvx59.dsl.pipex.com/Code%20of%20Practice%20booklet.pdf

Action-for-Advocacy. (2006b). *Quality standards for Advocacy schemes*. 2007, from http://www.aqvx59.dsl.pipex.com/Quality%20Standards%20Doc.pdf

Action-for-Advocacy. (2008). *Quality performance mark*. Retrieved October 3, 2008, from http://www.actionforadvocacy.org.uk/articleServlet?action=list&articletype=44

Action-for-Advocacy. (2009). Unit 305 independent mental capacity Advocacy – Skills, knowledge & competence.

Action-for-Advocacy. (2010). IMCA report writing best practice guidance [Electronic Version].

Action-for-Advocacy. (2011). The involvement of independent mental capacity advocates (IMCAs) in serious medical treatment decisions best practice guidance for healthcare professionals and IMCAs [Electronic Version], 1–74. Retrieved March 25, 2011, from http://static.actionforadvocacy.org.uk/opendocs/A4A_SMT_best_practice_guidance%282%29.pdf

Allen, R. (2012). The bluffers guide to healthcare chaplaincy. In *Newsletter of the Mental Health Resource Group*. London: College of Healthcare Chaplains.

© The Author(s) 2017

G. Morgan, *Independent Advocacy and Spiritual Care*,
DOI 10.1057/978-1-137-53125-4

Anandarajah, G., & Hight, E. (2001). Spirituality and medical practice: Using the HOPE questions as a practical tool for spiritual assessment. *American family physician, 63*(1), 81–89.

Angela, Y. (2007, October 1). Interviewer: G.Morgan, Advocacy interviews, Ivs-AY. London.

Anonymous. (2011). Health and well-being boards are given new scrutiny role [Electronic Version]. *Health Service Journal.* Retrieved December, 17, 2011, from http://www.hsj.co.uk/news/policy/health-and-wellbeing-boards-are--given-new-scrutiny-role/5023350.article

Anscombe, G. E. M. (1981). *The collected philosophical papers of G.E.M. Anscombe.* Minneapolis: University of Minnesota Press.

Archer, M., Bhaskar, R., Collier, A., Lawson, T., & Norrie, A. (Eds.). (1998). *Critical realism: Essential readings.* London/New York: Routledge.

Aristotle, Thomson, J. A. K., & Tredennick, H. (1976). *The ethics of Aristotle: The nicomachean ethics.* Harmondsworth/New York: Penguin.

Arnd-Caddigan, M., & Pozzuto, R. (2008). Use of self in relational clinical social work. *Clinical Social Work Journal, 36*(3), 235–243.

Aten, J. D., O'Grady, K. A., & Worthington, E. L. (Eds.). (2011). *The psychology of religion and spirituality for clinicians : Using research in your practice.* New York: Routledge.

Athanassoulis, N. (2006). Virtue [Electronic Version]. *The internet encyclopedia of philosophy.* Retrieved February 9, 2008, from http://www.iep.utm.edu/virtue/

Atkinson, D. (1999). *Advocacy- a review.* London: Pavilion/Joseph Rowntree.

Ballard, P. H. (1986). *The foundations of pastoral studies and practical theology.* Cardiff: Board of Studies for Pastoral Studies, University College.

Ballard, P. H. (2000). The emergence of pastoral and practical theology in Britain. In J. Woodward & S. Pattison (Eds.), *The Blackwell reader in pastoral and practical theology* (pp. 59–72). Oxford: Blackwell.

Ballard, P. H., & Pritchard, J. (1996). *Practical theology in action: Christian thinking in the service of church and society.* London: SPCK.

Barnes, D. (2006). Public communication, National Advocacy Policy Forum. In A. f. A. f. A. National Advocacy Policy Forum, 2006 (Ed.). Sheffield: Morgan, G.

Barnes, H. (Writer) (2011). The report, 24-11-2011, 20.00, BBC Radio 4: Deprivation of Liberty Safeguards, *The Report.*

Barnes, M., & Bowl, R. (2000). *Taking over the Asylum: Empowerment and mental health.* London/New York: Palgrave.

Barnes, D., Tate, A., & University of Durham. (2000). *Advocacy from the outside inside: A review of the patients' advocacy service at Ashworth Hospital.* Durham: University of Durham.

Barnum, B. S. (Ed.). (2011). *Spirituality in nursing: The challenges of complexity* (3rd ed.). New York: Springer.

Barrett, C. K. (1971). *A commentary on the first epistle to the corinthians.* London: A. & C. Black.

Bartlett, P. (1998). The asylum, the workhouse, and the voice of the insane poor in 19th-century England. *International Journal of Law and Psychiatry, 21*(4), 421–432.

Bateman, N. (2000). *Advocacy skills for health and social care professionals.* London/Philadelphia: J. Kingsley.

Batty, D. (2008, March 10). A scandal waiting to happen. *guardian.co.uk*

BBC-News. (2009, April 8). Church should fund NHS chaplains Retrieved April 23, 2009, from http://news.bbc.co.uk/1/hi/health/7988476.stm

BBC-News. (2011). Fiona Pilkington officers face misconduct proceedings [Electronic Version]. Retrieved September 30, 2012, from http://www.bbc.co.uk/news/uk-england-leicestershire-13504618

Beart, S., Hardy, G., & Buchan, L. (2004). Changing selves: A grounded theory account of belonging to a self-advocacy group for people with intellectual disabilities. *Journal of Applied Research in Intellectual Disabilities, 17*(2), 91–100.

Becker, H. S. (1961). *Boys in white; Student culture in medical school.* Chicago: University of Chicago Press.

Bella, B. (2010). Personal Communication. In G. Morgan (Ed.). London.

Bellamy, C., Jarrett, N., Mowbray, O., MacFarlane, P., Mowbray, C., & Holter, M. (2007). Relevance of spirituality for people with mental illness attending consumer-centered services. *Psychiatric Rehabilitation Journal, 30*(4), 287–294.

Bennett, Z. (2012). Britain. In B. J. Miller-McLemore (Ed.), *The Wiley-Blackwell companion to practical theology* (pp. 475–484). Malden: Wiley-Blackwell.

Beresford, P. (2007). *The changing roles and tasks of social work from service users' perspectives: A literature informed discussion paper.* London: Shaping Our Lives/General Social Care Council.

Beresford, P., Croft, S., & Adshead, L. (2008). 'We don't see her as a social worker': A service user case study of the importance of the social worker's relationship and humanity. *British Journal of Social Work, 38*(7), 1388–1407.

Bernard, A. (2008, August 19). Interviewer: G.Morgan, Advocacy interviews, Ivs-BA London.

Bertram, M. (2002). User involvement and mental health: Critical reflections on critical issues [Electronic Version]. *Psychminded, December 15th 2002.* Retrieved November 8, 2008, from http://www.psychminded.co.uk/news/news2002/1202/User%20Involvement%20and%20mental%20health%20reflections%20on%20critical%20issues.htm

Bhaskar, R. (2002a). The philosophy of meta-reality, part I: Identity, spirituality, system. interview by Mervyn Hartwig. *Journal of Critical Realism (Alethia), 1*(1), 67–93.

Bhaskar, R. (2002b). The philosophy of meta-reality, part II: Agency, perfectability, novelty. interview by Mervyn Hartwig. *Jounal of Critical Realism (Alethia), 1*(1), 21–34.

Bolton, G. (2005). *Reflective practice: Writing and professional development.* London/Thousand Oaks: Sage.

Bowes, A., & Sim, D. (2006). Advocacy for black and minority ethnic communities: Understandings and expectations. *British Journal of Social Work, 36*(7), 1209–1225.

Bowl, R. (1996). Legislating for user involvement in the United Kingdom: Mental health services and the NHS and Community Care Act 1990. *International ournal of social psychiatry, Autumn, 42*(3), 165–180.

Boyle, L. E. (1982). *The setting of the Summa theologiae of Saint Thomas.* Toronto, Ont., Canada: Pontifical Institute of Mediaeval Studies.

Bradshaw, A. (1994). *Lighting the lamp: The spiritual dimension of nursing care.* Harrow: Scutari Press.

Bradshaw, A. (2004). Changing perceptions of nurses' professional responsibility and lessons from history: A view from the United Kingdom. In B. Cusveller, A. Sutton, & D. O'Mathuna (Eds.), *Commitment and responsibility in nursing.* Iowa: Dordt College Press.

Bradshaw, P. L. (2008). Service user involvement in the NHS in England: Genuine user participation or a dogma-driven folly? *Journal of Nursing Management, 16*(6), 673–681.

Bradshaw, A. (2009). Measuring nursing care and compassion: The McDonaldised nurse? *Journal of medical ethics., 35,* 465–468.

Bradshaw, A. (2011). Care and compassion in nursing: Reflections from nursing history. *Nursing Times, 107*(19/20), 12–14.

Brandon, D. (1991). *Innovation without change?: Consumer power in psychiatric services.* Houndmills/Basingstoke/Hampshire: Macmillan.

Brandon, D. (2007). A friend to alleged lunatics. *Mental Health Today, 37*(9), 37–39.

Brandon, D., & Brandon, T. (2000). The history of advocacy in mental health. *Mental Health Practice, 3*(6), 6–8.

Bretherton, L. (2006). *Hospitality as holiness: Christian witness amid moral diversity.* Aldershot: Ashgate.

Brown, R. E. (1971). *Anchor Bible. Vol.29, The Gospel according to John, I-XII.* London: G. Chapman.

Brown, M. (2007). Spiritual advocacy. *Nursing Standard, 22*(13), 24–25.

Brown, J., & Libberton, P. (2007). *Principles of professional studies in nursing.* Basingstoke: Palgrave Macmillan.

Browning, D. S. (1991). *A fundamental practical theology: Descriptive and strategic proposals.* Minneapolis: Fortress Press.

Bruce, F. F. (1964). *The Epistle to the ebrews: The nglish text with introduction, exposition, and notes.* Grand Rapids: Wm. B. Eerdmans Pub. Co..

Campbell, P. (2001). The role of users of psychiatric services in service development – Influence not power. *Psychiatr Bull, 25*(3), 87–88.

Carver, N., & Morrison, J. (2005). Advocacy in practice: The experiences of independent advocates on UK mental health wards. *Journal of Psychiatric & Mental Health Nursing, 12*(1), 75–84.

Chappell, T. (2013). Virtue ethics in the twentieth century. In D. Russell (Ed.), *The Cambridge companion to virtue ethics* (pp. 149–171). Cambridge/New York: Cambridge University Press.

Charlton, J. I. (1998). *Nothing about us without us: Disability oppression and empowerment.* Berkeley: University of California Press.

Cobb, M. (2004). The location and identity of chaplains: A contextual model. *Scottish Journal of Healthcare Chaplaincy, 7*(2), 10–14.

Cochrane, S. e. (2003). *SPN Paper 4: Where you stand affects your point of view. Emancipatory approaches to mental health research Notes from SPN Study Day: 12 June 2003*, London.

Commons, H. o. (2011). *Disability: Advocacy Written answers and statements, 16th May 2011.* Retrieved May 22, 2011, from http://www.publications.parliament.uk/pa/cm201011/cmhansrd/cm110516/text/110516w0003.htm#11051625001570

Commons, H. o. (2014). *Valuing every voice, respecting every right: Making the case for the Mental Capacity Act. The Government's response to the House of Lords Select Committee*, London.

Community-Services-Improvement-Partnership/London-Development-Council. (2007, October 25). *BME Advocacy and the Mental Health Act.*

Copsey, N. (1997). *Keeping faith: The provision of community mental health services within a multi-faith context.* London: Sainsbury Centre for Mental Health.

Copsey, N. (2012, June 14) *Spiritual care.* Paper presented at the National Spirituality and Menta Health Forum, London.

Cornah, D. (2006). *The impact of spirituality on mental health. A literature review.* London: Mental Health Foundation.

Cornwell, J. (1984). *Hard-earned lives: Accounts of health and illness from East London.* London/New York: Tavistock Publications/Methuen.

Cox, J., Campbell, A. V., & Fulford, K. W. M. (Eds.). (2007). *Medicine of the person: Faith, science and values in health care provision.* London: Jessica Kingsley.

Coyle, M. (2008). *Here for good? A snapshot of the advocacy workforce.* London: Action-for-Advocacy.

Coyle, M. (2010). Email. In G. Morgan (Ed.). Leeds.

Coyle, M. (2013). Demand for advocacy is rising as funding and access fall [Electronic Version]. *Guardian, social care network: Adult social care hub.* Retrieved October 13, 2015, from http://www.theguardian.com/social-care-network/2013/sep/04/demand-for-advocacy-rising

Coyte, M. E., Gilbert, P., & Nicholls, V. (Eds.). (2008). *Spirituality, values, and mental health: Jewels for the journey.* London/Philadelphia: Jessica Kingsley Publishers.

Creswell, J. W. (2009). *Research design: Qualitative, quantitative, and mixed methods approaches.* Los Angeles: Sage.

Cribb, A., & Duncan, P. (2002). *Health promotion and professional ethics.* Oxford: Blackwell.

Croft, S., & Beresford, P. (1989). User-involvement, citizenship and social policy. *Critical Social Policy, 9*(26), 5–18.

Croft, S., & Beresford, P. (1992). The politics of participation. *Critical Social Policy, 12*(35), 20–44.

Crossley, N. (1999). Fish, field, habitus and madness: The first wave mental health users movement in Great Britain*. *The British Journal of Sociology, 50*(4), 647–670.

Crossley, N. (2007). Social networks and extraparliamentary politics. *Sociology Compass, 1*(1), 222–236.

Crossley, N, & NetLibrary, I. (2006). *Contesting psychiatry social movements in mental health.* London: Routledge.

Culliford, L. (2010). *The psychology of spirituality: An introduction.* London/Philadelphia: Jessica Kingsley Publishers.

Culliford, L., & Powell, A. (2006). *Help is at hand: Spirituality and mental health.* London: Royal College of Psychiatrists' Spirituality and Psychiatry Special Interest Group.

Dalrymple, J. (2004). Developing the concept of professional advocacy: An examination of the role of child and youth advocates in England and wales. *Journal of Social Work, 4*(2), 179–197.

Dalton, S., & Carlin, P. (2002). Independent advocacy – A brief look at its past and present – Is its future under threat. *Journal of Mental Health Law, 21*, 21–34.

Darwall, S. L. (2002). *Virtue ethics.* Oxford: Blackwell.

Davies, C. A. (1999). *Reflexive ethnography: A guide to researching selves and others.* London: Routledge.

Delany, J. (1911). Corporal and spiritual works of mercy [Electronic Version]. *The Catholic Encyclopedia* Retrieved September 3, 2010, from New Advent: http://www.newadvent.org/cathen/10198d.htm

Department-of-Health. (2013). *Post-legislative Scrutiny of the Mental Health Act 2007: Response to the report of the health committee of the house of commons.* Retrieved October 13, 2015, from https://www.gov.uk/government/uploads/system/uploads/attachment_data/file/252876/33736_Cm_8735_Web_Accessible.pdf

Department-of-Health. (2014). *The seventh year of the independent mental capacity Advocacy (IMCA) service.* London.

Department-of-Health-and-the-Welsh-Assembly. (2008). The Award Project. Retrieved October 9, 2008, from http://www.nimhe.csip.org.uk/~advocacy

Dept.-for-Constitutional-Affairs. (2006a). *Human rights: Human lives: a handbook for public authorities.* London: Department for Constitutional Affairs.

Dept.-for-Constitutional-Affairs. (2006b). *Mental capacity act code of practice.* London: Department for Constitutional Affairs.

Dept.-of-Health. (2010a). *A vision for adult social care: Capable communities and active citizens.* London: Social Care Policy Department.

Dept-of-Health. (2010b). *The third year of the independent mental Capacity Advocacy (IMCA) service 2009–10.* Retrieved May 24, 2011, from http://www.dh.gov.uk/en/Publicationsandstatistics/Publications/PublicationsPolicyAndGuidance/DH_121877

Dimond, L. (2003). Independent complaints advocacy services for patients (ICAS). *Clin Risk, 9*(2), 69–71.

Diwan, S. (2015, September 11). *College of healthcare chaplains conference, plenary session.* Paper presented at the Pilgrims in a New Land- working in a world of transformation, High Leigh Conference Centre.

DoH. (1990). *The NHS and community care act.* London: HMSO.

(DoH, D. o. H.). (1995). *Consumers and research in the NHS.* Leeds.

DoH. (2001). *Valuing people. A new strategy for learning disability for the 21st century*. London: Department of Health.

DoH. (2006). *Our health, our care, our say. A new direction for community services*. London: TSO.

DoH. (2007). *Putting people first: A shared vision and commitment to the transformation of adult social care*. London: TSO.

(DoH). (2008a). Independent Mental Capacity Act (IMCA) Service. from http://www.dh.gov.uk/en/SocialCare/Deliveringadultsocialcare/MentalCapacity/IMCA/DH_4135239

DoH. (2008b). *Mental capacity act 2005 deprivation of liberty safeguards in England*. London: Department of Health.

DoH. (2008c). *Transforming social care, LAC (DH) (2008) 1, 17*. London: TSO.

DoH. (2008d). *The future regulation of health and adult social care in England: A consultation on the framework for the registration of health and adult social care providers*. London: TSO.

(DoH). (2009). *Good learning disability partnership boards: 'Making it happen for everyone'*.

(DoH). (2013). *Independent mental capacity advocacy service – Fifth annual report*. London.

(DoH, & The-British-Institute-of-Human-Rights). (2007). *Human rights in healthcare- a framework for local action*.

Doherty, D. (2006). Spirituality and dementia. *Spirituality and Health International, 7*(4), 203–210.

Dorothy, W. (2008, September 18). Interviewer: G.Morgan, Advocacy interviews, Ivs-DW. London.

Duncan, P. (2002). *Local authorities and the 'Power of Well-Being'*. Centre for public policy research, King's College London.

Dunn, M. C., Clare, I. C. H., Holland, A. J., & Gunn, M. J. (2007). Constructing and reconstructing 'Best Interests': An interpretative examination of substitute decision-making under the mental capacity act 2005. *Journal of Social Welfare and Family Law, 29*(2), 117–133.

Dunning, A., & Joseph Rowntree, F. (2005). *Information, advice and advocacy for older people: Defining and developing services*. York: Joseph Rowntree Foundation.

Eagger, S. (2005a). A short guide to the assessment of spiritual concerns in mental healthcare [Electronic Version]. Retrieved March 27, 2011, from http://www.rcpsych.ac.uk/PDF/DrSEaggeGuide.pdf

Eagger, S. (2005b). Spirituality and the practice of healthcare: Robinson, S., Kendrick, K., Brown A. Basingstoke: Palgrave. *Psychiatr Bull, 29*(3), 118-a.

Eisikovits, Z., & Beker, J. (2001). Beyond professionalism: The child and youth care worker as craftsman. *Child and Youth Care Forum, 30*(6), 415–434.

El Ansari, W., Newbigging, K. A., Roth, C., & Malik, F. (2009). The role of advocacy and interpretation services in the delivery of quality healthcare to diverse minority communities in London, United Kingdom. *Health & Social Care in the Community, 17*(6), 636–646.

Ely, M., & Anzul, M. (Eds.). (1991). *Doing qualitative research: Circles within circles.* London: Falmer Press.

Emerson, E., Robertson, J., Gregory, N., Kessissoglou, S., Hatton, C., Hallam, A., et al. (2000). The quality and costs of community-based residential supports and residential campuses for people with severe and complex disabilities. *Journal of Intellectual & Developmental Disability, 25*(4), 263–279.

Eraut, M. (1994). *Developing professional knowledge and competence.* London/Washington, D.C.: Falmer Press.

Eraut, M. (2000). Non-formal learning and tacit knowledge in professional work. *British journal of educational psychology, 70,* 113–136.

Eraut, M. (2004). Informal learning in the workplace. *Studies in Continuing Education, 26*(2), 247–273.

Evans, S. M. (1979). *Personal politics: The roots of women's liberation in the civil rights movement and the new left.* New York: Knopf: distributed by Random House. [2011] EWHC (England & Wales High Court) 1377 (COP) [Court of Protection] (2011).

Fairbank, J. K, Twitchett, D. C, & Mote, F. W. (1998). *The Cambridge history of China. Vol. 8, The Ming dynasty, 1368–1644* (p. 2). Cambridge: Cambridge Univ. Press.

Farley, E. (1983). Theology and practice outside the clerical paradigm. In D. S. Browning & J. E. Burkhart (Eds.), *Practical theology: The emerging field in theology, church, and world* (pp. 21–41). San Francisco [u.a.]: Harper & Row.

Faust, J. (2008). Clinical social worker as patient advocate in a community mental health center. *Clinical Social Work Journal, 36*(3), 293–300.

Fauzia, B. (2007, October 1). Interviewer: G.Morgan, Advocacy interviews, Ivs-FB London.

Fielding, M. (1996). Empowerment: Emancipation or enervation? *Journal of Education Policy, 11*(3), 399–417.

Flanagan, K., & Davie, G. (1995). Review of religion in Britain since 1945. Believing without belonging. *British Journal of Sociology, 46*(4), 742.

Foley, R., & Platzer, H. (2007). Place and provision: Mapping mental health advocacy services in London. *Social Science & Medicine, 64*(3), 617–632.

Forbat, L., & Atkinson, D. (2005). Advocacy in practice: The troubled position of advocates in adult Services. *British Journal of Social Work, 35*(3), 321–335.

Forster, R. (1998). Patient advocacy in psychiatry: The Austrian and the Dutch models. *International Social Work, 41*(2), 155–167.

Foskett, J. (2004). Editorial. *Mental Health, Religion & Culture, 7*(1), 1–3.

Foskett, J., Marriott, J., & Wilson-Rudd, F. (2004a). Mental health, religion and spirituality: Attitudes, experience and expertise among mental health professionals and religious leaders in somerset. *Mental Health, Religion & Culture, 7*(1), 5–22.

Foskett, J., Roberts, A., Mathews, R., Macmin, L., Cracknell, P., & Nicholls, V. (2004b). From research to practice: The first tentative steps. *Mental Health, Religion & Culture, 7*(1), 41–58.

Foucault, M. (1967). *Madness and civilization: A history of insanity in the age of reason.* London: Routledge.

Freeman, J. (1975). *The Politics of women's liberation: A case study of an emerging social movement and its relation to the policy process.* New York: David McKay.

Freeman, H. (1998). Mental health policy and practice in the NHS: 1948–79. *Journal of Mental Health, 7*, 225–239.

Fulford, K., Ersser, S., & Hope, T. (Eds.). (1996). *Essential practice in patient-centred care.* Oxford: Blackwell Science.

Funk, M., Minoletti, A., Drew, N., Taylor, J., & Saraceno, B. (2006). Advocacy for mental health: Roles for consumer and family organizations and governments. *Health Promot. Int., 21*(1), 70–75.

Furbey, R., & Joseph Rowntree, F. (2006). *Faith as social capital: Connecting or dividing?* Bristol: Policy Press.

Gamble, D. (1999). The value of advocacy: Putting ethics in to practice. *Psychiatr Bull, 23*(9), 569-b-570.

Gammack, G. (2011a). *Advocacy and exodus- from Moses to the mental health act.* London: Spiderwize.

Gammack, G. (2011b). email. In G. Morgan (Ed.). London.

Gammell, C. (2009, February 7). Nurse Caroline Petrie: I will continue praying for patients. *The Daily Telegraph.* Retrieved April 23, 2009, from http://www.telegraph.co.uk/news/newstopics/religion/4537452/Nurse-Caroline-Petrie-I-will-continue-praying-for-patients.html

Gates, B. (2002). *Learning disabilities.* Edinburgh: Churchill Livingstone.

Gault, H. (2008). An expert by experience. *The Psychologist, 21*(5), 462–463.

Gaventa, W. C., & Coulter, D. L. (2001). *The theological voice of wolf wolfensberger.* New York: Haworth Pastoral Press.

Geach, P. (1977). *The virtues: The stanton lectures 1973–4*. Cambridge: University Press.

Giddens, A. (1991). *Modernity and self-identity: Self and society in the late modern age*. Stanford: Stanford University Press.

Giddens, A., & Birdsall, K. (2001). *Sociology*. Cambridge [England]: Polity Press.

Gilbert, P. (2007a). Framework for the mental health and spirituality project Pilot Sites. London: unpublished email.

Gilbert, P. (2007b). Framework for the mental health and spirituality project Pilot Sites, unpublished email. In G. Morgan (Ed.). London: unpublished email.

Gilbert, P. (2008). Nurturing a new discourse: Mental health and spirituality. *Spirituality and Health International*, n/a.

Gilbert, P. (2010). Seeking inspiration: The rediscovery of the spiritual dimension in health and social care in England. *Mental Health, Religion & Culture*, *13*(1), 1–14.

Gilbert, P. (Ed.). (2011). *Spirituality and mental health: A handbook for service users, carers and staff wishing to bring a spiritual dimension to mental health services*. Brighton: Pavilion.

Gilbert, P., & Nicholls, V. (2003). *Inspiring hope: Recognising the importance of spirituality in a whole person approach to mental health*. Leeds: NIMHE.

Gilbert, P., Persaud, A., & Hawes, A. (2006). *SPN paper 9: Reaching the spirit. Spirituality and mental health notes from study day: April 4th 2006*. Paper presented at the Social Perspectives Network.

Gill, R. (2001). *The Cambridge companion to Christian ethics*. Cambridge, U.K./ New York: Cambridge University Press.

Glynn, T. (2003). There is a better way. In S. Cochrane (Ed.), *SPN paper 4: Where you stand affects your point of view. Emancipatory approaches to mental health research notes from SPN study day: 12 June 2003* (pp. 64–66). London: Social Perspectives Network.

Gorczynska, T. (2007). The first legal right to advocacy. *Working with older people: Community care policy & practice*, *11*(1), 17–20.

Gorczynska, T., & Thompson, D. (2007). The role of the independent mental capacity advocate in adult protection. *The Journal of Adult Protection*, *9*(4), 38–45.

Graham, E. (2010). The 'virtuous circle'. Religion and the practices of happiness. In I. Steedman (Ed.), *The practices of happiness* (pp. 224–234). London: Taylor and Francis.

Graham, M. (2015). *A practical guide to the mental capacity act 2005: Putting the principles of the act into practice*. London: Jessica Kingsley Publishers.

Gramsci, A., Hoare, Q., & Nowell-Smith, G. (1972). *Selections from the prison notebooks of Antonio Gramsci*. New York: International Publishers.

Grant, G. (2005). *Learning disability: A life cycle approach to valuing people*. Maidenhead/New York: Open University Press.

Green, M., & Christian, C. (1998). *Accompanying young people on their spiritual quest*. London: National Society/Church House Pub.

Griffin, A. P. (1983). A philosophical analysis of caring in nursing. *Journal of advanced nursing, 8*(4), 289–295.

Grover, S. (2004). Advocating for children's rights as an aspect of professionalism: The role of frontline workers and children's rights commissions. *Child & Youth Care Forum, 33*(6), 405–423.

Habib, C. (2007, October 1). Interviewer: G.Morgan, Advocacy interviews, Ivs-HC London.

Hampshire-County-Council. (2008). Putting people first – shaping your future, choosing your care. Commission of Inquiry into the future services for adults in need of support and care. Retrieved November 27, 2008, from http://www3.hants.gov.uk/adult-services/aboutas/consultation-involvement/commission-personalisation.htm

Harlow, R. (2010). Developing a spirituality strategy – Why, how, and so what? *Mental Health, Religion and Culture, 13*(6), 615–624.

Harrison, G. (2011). *The spiritual and pastoral care of service users, Standard Operating Procedure (SOP)*. West London Mental Health NHS Trust.

Harrison, T., & Davis, R. (2009). Advocacy: Time to communicate. *Advances in Psychiatric Treamentt, 15*(1), 57–64.

Haslam, J., & Porter, R. (1988). *Illustrations of madness*. London/New York: Routledge.

Hauerwas, S. (1993). *Naming the silences: God, medicine, and the problem of suffering*. Edinburgh: T. & T. Clark.

Hauerwas, S., & Berkman, J. (2005). *The Hauerwas reader*. Durham [u.a.]: Duke Univ. Press.

Heelas, P., & Woodhead, L. (2007). *The spiritual revolution: Why religion is giving way to spirituality*. Malden, MA: Blackwell.

Helminiak, D. A. (2006). The role of spirituality in formulating a theory of the psychology of religion. *Zygon®, 41*(1), 197–224.

Henderson, R. (2005). Mental health advocacy and empowerment in focus. In T. Ryan, J. Pritchard, et al. (Eds.), *Good practice in adult mental health* (pp. 202–215). London/Philadelphia: Jessica Kingsley Publishers.

Henderson, R. (2007). Award for all? *Planet advocacy, June-August 2007*, 16–17.

Henderson, R., & Pochin, M. (2001). *A right result?: Advocacy, justice and empowerment*. Bristol: Policy.

Hervey, N. (1986). Advocacy or folly: The alleged lunatics' friend society, 1845–63. *Med Hist., 30*(3), 245–275.

Hospital-Chaplaincies-Council. (2010). *Health care chaplaincy and the church of England, a review of the work of the Hospital Chaplaincies Council*. London: Church of England.

Hunter, B., & Deery, R. (2009). *Emotions in midwifery and reproduction*. Basingstoke/New York: Palgrave Macmillan.

Jana, D. (2007, October 22). Interviewer: G.Morgan, Advocacy interviews, Ivs-JD. London.

Janine, E. (2007, October 1). Interviewer: G.Morgan, Advocacy interviews, Ivs-JE. London.

Jarvis, P. (1999). *The practitioner-researcher: Developing theory from practice*. San Francisco: Jossey-Bass.

Jewell, A., & Kitwood, T. (Eds.). (2011). *Spirituality, personhood, and dementia*. Philadelphia: Jessica Kingsley Publishers.

Johnson, T. J. (1972). *Professions and power*. London: Macmillan.

Johnson, S., & Harlow, R. (2011). *The role of the Spiritual Advocate: Emerging ideas, A paper prepared by Stuart Johnson, with additional material by Richard Harlow*: Sussex Partnership NHS Trust.

Jones, K. (1972). *A history of the mental health services*. London/Boston: Routledge and Kegan Paul.

Jordan, M. D. (1986). *Ordering wisdom: The hierarchy of philosophical discourses in Aquinas*. Notre Dame: University of Notre Dame Press.

Karban, K. (2011). *Social work and mental health*. Cambridge: Polity Press.

Kelly, E. (2013). *Personhood and presence: Self as a resource for spiritual and pastoral care*. London: Bloomsbury.

Kerr, F. (2002). *After aquinas: Versions of thomism*. Malden: Blackwell Publishers.

Kevin, W. (2008, January 14). Interviewer: G.Morgan, Advocacy interviews, Ivs-KW. London.

Klein, R., & Millar, J. (1995). Do-it-yourself social policy: Searching for a new paradigm? *Social Policy & Administration, 29*(4), 303–316.

Klijnsma, M. P. (1993). Patient advocacy in the Netherlands. *Psychiatr Bull, 17*(4), 230–231.

Knight, K. (Ed.). (1998). *The macintyre reader*. Oxford: Polity Press.

Knight, P. (2011). *Determining the attitudes of mental health professionals toward integrating spirituality*. unknown: unknown.

Koehn, D. (1994). *The ground of professional ethics*. London/New York: Routlege.

Koenig, H., & Larson, D. (2001). Religion and mental health: Evidence for an association. *International Review of Psychiatry, 13*(2), 67–78.

Layard, R. (2007). *The teaching of values*. Paper presented at the The 2007 Ashby Lecture.

Layard, R. (2009, September 14). This is the greatest good. We have only one true yardstick with which to measure society's progress: Happiness. *The Guardian*, 32.

Legislation.gov.uk. (2012). Health and Social Care Act [Electronic Version] from http://www.legislation.gov.uk/ukpga/2012/7/section/185/enacted

Legislation.gov.uk. (2014). Health and Social Care Act [Electronic Version]. Retrieved September 22, 2015, from http://www.legislation.gov.uk/ukpga/2014/23/section/67/enacted

Lewis, C. S. (1952, February 8). Letters. *Church Times*.

Lewis, P. W. (1998). A pneumatolgical approach to virtue ethics. *Asian Journal of Pentecostal Studies, 1*(1).

Little, W., Fowler, H. W., Coulson, J., Onions, C. T., & Friedrichsen, G. W. S. (1983). *The shorter oxford english dictionary on historical principles*. London: Book Club Associates.

Llewellyn, P., & Northway, R. (2007). The views and experiences of learning disability nurses concerning their advocacy education. *Nurse Education Today, 27*(8), 955–963.

Louise, F., Michael, G., Pixy, H., Whitney, I., & Germaine, G. (2007, November 23). Interviewer: G.Morgan, Advocacy interviews, Ivs-LF et al. London.

Luke, L., Redley, M., Clare, I., & Holland, A. (2008). Hospital clinicians' attitudes towards a statutory advocacy service for patients lacking mental capacity: Implications for implementation. *Journal of Health Service Research Policy, 13*(2), 73–78.

Lyall, D. (1995). *Counselling in the pastoral and spiritual context*. In *Buckingham*. Philadelphia: Open University Press.

Lyall, D. (2010). *Pastoral care and counselling in Scotland since 1950*. Paper presented at the theology and therapy conference.

MacDonald, H. (2007). Relational ethics and advocacy in nursing: Literature review. *Journal of Advanced Nursing, 57*(2), 119–126.

MacIntyre, A. C. (1985). *After virtue: A study in moral theory*. London: Duckworth.

MacIntyre, A. C. (1988). *Whose justice? Which rationality?* Notre Dame: University of Notre Dame Press.

MacIntyre, A. C. (1990). *Three rival versions of moral enquiry: Encyclopaedia, genealogy, and tradition: Being Gifford lectures delivered in the University of Edinburgh in 1988*. Notre Dame: University of Notre Dame Press.

MacIntyre, A. C. (1999). *Dependent rational animals: Why human beings need the virtues*. London: Duckworth.

Mackey, R. (2008). Toward an integration of ideas about the self for the practice of clinical social work. *Clinical Social Work Journal, 36*(3), 225–234.

Macmin, L., & Foskett, J. (2004). "Don't be afraid to tell." The spiritual and religious experience of mental health service users in somerset. *Mental Health, Religion & Culture, 7*(1), 23–40.

Maddox, R. (1991). Practical theology: A discipline in search of a definition. *Perspectives in Religious Studies, 18*, 159–169.

Mallik, M. (1997). Advocacy in nursing – A review of the literature. *Journal of Advanced Nursing, 25*(1), 130–138.

Mallik, M. (1998). Advocacy in nursing: Perceptions and attitudes of the nursing elite in the United Kingdom. *Journal of Advanced Nursing, 28*(5), 1001–1011.

Mallik, M., & Rafferty, A. M. (2000). Diffusion of the concept of patient advocacy. *Journal of Nursing Scholarship, 32*(4), 399–404.

Maltby, J., Lewis, C. A., & Day, L. (2008). Prayer and subjective well-being: The application of a cognitive-behavioural framework. *Mental Health, Religion & Culture, 11*(1), 119–129.

Maria, M. (2007, October 1). Interviewer: G.Morgan, Advocacy interviews, Ivs-MM. London.

Marshall, T. H. (1973). *Class, citizenship, and social development; Essays*. Westport: Greenwood Press.

Martin, G. (2000). *Social movements of care, CAVA workshop paper 23*. Paper presented at the Prepared for Workshop Six: Cross National Perspectives and Issues.

Mason, J. (2002). *Researching your own practice: The discipline of noticing*. London: RoutledgeFalmer.

McKeown, M., Bingley, W., & Denoual, I. (2002). *Review of Advocacy Services at the Edenfield Regional Secure Unit and Bowness High Dependency Unit, Prestwich Hsopital*. Preston: University of Central Lancashire.

McKeown, M., Malihi-Shoja, L., & Downe, S. (2010). *Service user and carer involvement in education for health and social care*. Chichester/West Sussex/Ames/Iowa: Wiley-Blackwell.

McNiff, J. (2002). *Action research principles and practice*. London/New York: Routledge.

McSherry, W., & Jamieson, S. (2011). An online survey of nurses' perceptions of spirituality and spiritual care. *Journal of Clinical Nursing, 20*(11–12), 1757–1767.

McSherry, W., & Ross, L. (Eds.). (2010). *Spiritual assessment in healthcare practice*. Keswick: M & K.

McSherry, W., Gretton, M., Draper, P., & Watson, R. (2008). The ethical basis of teaching spirituality and spiritual care: A survey of student nurses perceptions. *Nurse Educ. Today Nurse Education Today, 28*(8), 1003–1009.

Mental-Health-Act-Commission. (2007). Mental Health Act 2007 Policy Briefing for Commissioners. Retrieved August 22, 2007.

Mercer, K. (2007). In T. Researcher (Ed.). London.

Metropolitan-Anthony-Bloom. (2012). On the cross of our lord. Retrieved October 9, 2012, from, http://www.stmaryorthodoxchurch.org/orthodoxy/quotes.php

Micky, K, Einstein, L, Yolanda, M, Norma, N, Robert, O, Madonna, P, et al. (2008, May 14). Interviewer: G.Morgan, Advocacy interviews, Ivs-MK et al. London.

Millar, J. (1996). Family obligations and social policy: The case of child support. *Policy Studies, 17*(3), 181–193.

Miller-McLemore, B. J. (2012). Introduction: The contributions of practical theology. In B. J. Miller-McLemore (Ed.), *The Wiley-Blackwell companion to practical theology* (pp. 1–20). Malden: Wiley-Blackwell.

MIND. (2008). MIND guide to advocacy. Retrieved November 1, 2008, from http://www.mind.org.uk/Information/Booklets/Mind+guide+to/advocacy.htm

Ministerial-Statement. (2007). Retrieved August 22, 2007, from http://www.publications.parliament.uk/pa/cm200607/cmhansrd/cm070423/wmstext/70423m0001.htm#0704237000001

Monro, J. (1758). *Remarks on Dr Battie's treatise on madness, by John Monro, M.D.* London: printed for John Clarke.

Morgan, G. (1997). *An analytical, critical and comparative study of Anglican mission in the dioceses of Nakuru and Mount Kenya East, Kenya, from 1975*. Unpublished M.Phil, Open, Oxford.

Morgan, G. (2010). Independent advocacy and the "rise of spirituality": Views from advocates, service users and chaplains. *Mental Health, Religion & Culture, 13*(6), 625–636.

Morgan, G. (2010). Meeting notes. Retrieved June 5, 2012, from http://mhspirituality.org.uk/meetingnotes.html

Morgan, G. (2011a). Independent advocacy, neuro-disability and spirituality? A history of advocacy with a case study from the independent mental capacity advocate (IMCA) service. *Social Care and Neurodisability, 2*(4), 208–217.

Morgan, G. (2011b). Spiritual advocacy in England? The overlapping roles of chaplains and advocates. In K. Chappell & F. Davis (Eds.), *Catholic social conscience: Reflection and action on catholic social teaching* (pp. 199–219). Leominster: Gracewing.

Morgan, G. (2014). *Spirit of Advocacy. Theory and practice in independent advocacy:an historical and qualitative analysis using Practical Theology.* Unpublished PhD, King's College London, London.

Morgan, G. (2015). Spiritual advocacy in England? How the overlapping roles of chaplains and independent advocates benefit the most vulnerable in society. In E. C. Roberts (Ed.), *Spirituality: Global practices, societal attitudes and effects on health.* New York: Nova Science.

NAN. (2007). http://www.advocacynetwork.org.uk/component/option,com_frontpage/Itemid,29/

Naughtie, J. (Writer) (2008). Interview with Lenny Harper, former Deputy Chief Officer, Jersey Police on enquiry at Haut de la Garenne children's home, Jersey [Radio], *Today Programme.* UK: BBC.

Nebi, S. (2007, October 22). Interviewer: G.Morgan, Advocacy interviews, Ivs-NS. London.

Newbigging, K. a., & McKeown, M. b. (2007). Mental health advocacy with black and minority ethnic communities: Conceptual and ethical implications. *Current Opinion in Psychiatry, 20*(6), 588–593.

Newbigging, R., McKeown, M., Poursanidou, A., et al. (2012). *The right to be heard review of the mental aealth Advocate (IMHA) services in England.* University of Central Lancashire.

Newbigging, K., Ridley, J., McKeown, M., Sadd, J., Machin, K., Cruse, K., et al. (2015). *Independent mental health advocacy – The right to be heard context, values and good practice.* London: Jessica Kingsley Publishers.

NHS Executive. (1996). *Patient partnership: Building a collaborative strategy.* Leeds: DoH.

Nigel, A, & Colin, B. (2008, September 11). Interviewer: G.Morgan, Advocacy interviews, Ivs-NA&CB. London.

Norah, A. (1990). Karen. Personal Communication in G.Morgan (Ed.), London.

Norah, A., & Bella, B. (2009, December 14). Interviewer: G.Morgan, Advocacy interviews Ivs-NA & BB. London.

Norman, A., & Colin, B. (2008, September 11). Interviewer: G.Morgan, Advocacy interviews, Ivs-NA/CB. London.

Northcott, M. S. (2003). Do dolphins carry the cross biological moral realism and theological ethics. *New Blackfriars, 84*(994), 540–553.

Nussbaum, M. C. (1986). *The fragility of goodness: Luck and ethics in Greek tragedy and philosophy*. Cambridge/New York: Cambridge University Press.

Oden, T. C. (1994). *Classical pastoral care*. Grand Rapids/Michigan: Baker Books.

Office-for-National-Statistics. (2012). *Measuring National Wellbeing*. Retrieved October 6, 2012, from http://www.ons.gov.uk/ons/guide-method/user-guidance/well-being/index.html

Older-People's-Advocacy-Alliance. (2008). http://www.opaal.org.uk/. Retrieved October 14, 2008, from http://www.opaal.org.uk/

Olive, P. (2007, November 7). Interviewer: G.Morgan, Advocacy interviews, Ivs-OP. London.

Oliver, M. (1990). *The politics of disablement: A sociological approach*. New York: St. Martin's Press.

Oliver, T. (2012, January Monday 16th – Friday 20th). *Chaplaincy and Ethics-End of Life*. Paper presented at the Training course for healthcare Chaplains, St Michael's Theological College, Cardiff.

Pargament, K. I. (2011). *Spiritually integrated psychotherapy: Understanding and addressing the sacred*. New York: Guilford.

Parry, O., Pithouse, A., Anglim, C., & Batchelor, C. (2008). 'The tip of the ice berg': Children's complaints and advocacy in Wales—An insider view from complaints officers. *British Journal of Social Work, 38*(1), 5–19.

Pattison, S. (Ed.). (1994). *Pastoral care and liberation theology*. Cambridge: Cambridge University Press.

Pattison, S. (2000). *A critique of pastoral care*. London: SCM Press.

Pattison, S. (2007a). Pastoral studies: Dust bin or discipline? In S. Pattison (Ed.), *The challenge of practical theology: Selected essays* (pp. 247–252). London/Philadelphia: Jessica Kingsley Publishers.

Pattison, S. (2007b). Practical theology: Art or science? In S. Pattison (Ed.), *The challenge of practical theology: Selected essays* (pp. 261–289). London/Philadelphia: Jessica Kingsley Publishers.

Pattison, S., & Woodward, J. (2000). An introduction to pastoral and practical theology. In J. W. a. S. Pattison (Ed.), *The Blackwell reader in pastoral and practical theology*. Oxford: Blackwell.

Payne, H., & Pithouse, A. (2006). More aspiration than achievement? Children's complaints and advocacy in health services in Wales. *Health & Social Care in the Community, 14*(6), 563–571.

Perceval, J., & Bateson, G. (1962). *Perceval's narrative: A patient's account of his psychosis*. London: Hogarth Press.

Pesut, B. P. R. N. (2008). A conversation on diverse perspectives of spirituality in nursing literature. *Nursing Philosophy, 9*(2), 98–109.

Peteet, J. R., & D'Ambra, M. N. (Eds.). (2011). *The soul of medicine: Spiritual perspectives and clinical practice*. Baltimore: Johns Hopkins University Press.

Peter, U. (2008, December 9). Interviewer: G.Morgan, Advocacy interviews, Ivs-PU. London.

Pilgrim, D., & Waldron, L. (1998). User involvement in mental health service development. How far can it go? *Journal of Mental Health, 7*(1), 95–104.

Pithouse, A., & Crowley, A. (2007). Adults rule? Children, advocacy and complaints to social services. *Children & Society, 21*(3), 201–213.

Porter, J. (2001). Virtue ethics. In R. Gill (Ed.), *The Cambridge companion to christian ethics* (pp. 87–102). Cambridge: Cambridge University Press.

Powell, A. (2011). *Opening remarks*. Paper presented at the Doctors, Clergy and the Troubled Soul, Marylebone/London.

Preface to volumes. (1986). World spirituality: An encyclopedic history of the religious quest (Ed.)^(Eds.). London: Routledge & Kegan Paul.

Prigg, M. (2010, February 24). Google bosses convicted over abuse video of Down's syndrome boy. *Evening Standard*.

Pritchard, J. (2009). *Good practice in the law and safeguarding adults: Criminal justice and adult protection*. London/Philadelphia: Jessica Kingsley Publishers.

Raffay, J. (2011). Assessing spiritual strengths and needs [Electronic Version]. *The Journal of Healthcare Chaplaincy, 11*, 50–64 from http://www.health-carechaplains.org/information/documents/journal_spring_2011.pdf.

Rai-Atkins, A. (2002). *Best practice in mental health: Advocacy for African, Caribbean, and South Asian communities*. Bristol: Published for the Joseph Rowntree Foundation by Policy Press.

Ramcharan, P., & Grant, G. (2001). Views and experiences of people with intellectual disabilities and their families. (1) The user perspective. *Journal of Applied Research in Intellectual Disabilities, 14*(4), 348–363.

Ravich, R., & Schmolka, L. (1996). Patient representation: A patient-centred approach to the provision of health services. In K. Fulford, S. Ersser, & T. Hope (Eds.), *Essential practice in patient-centred care* (pp. 68–85). Oxford: Blackwell.

Rawls, J. (1971). *A theory of justice*. Cambridge, MA: Belknap Press of Harvard University Press.

Rawls, J. (1999). *The law of peoples; With, the idea of public reason revisited.* Cambridge, MA: Harvard University Press.

RCPsych. (2008). Publication. Retrieved June 2, 2008, from Royal College of Psychiatrists http://www.rcpsych.ac.uk/college/specialinterestgroups/spirituality.aspx

Reinders, H. S. (2007). In conversation with Hans Ulrich's Wie Geschopfe Leben. *Studies in Christian Ethics, 20*(2), 231–256.

Reinders, H. S. (2008). Persons with disabilities as parents: What is the problem? *Journal of Applied Research in Intellectual Disabilities, 21*(4), 308–314.

Riches, C. (2010, March 12). A 'true gent' tormented to death by gang of yobs. *Daily Express.*

Ridley, J., & Jones, L. (2001). *User and public involvement in health services: A literature review.* Edinburgh: Partners in Change.

Roberts, A. (1981a). Mental health history timeline from http://www.mdx.ac.uk/www/study/mhhtim.htm

Roberts, A. (1981b). *The Lunacy Commission: A study of its origin, emergence and character.* Retrieved November 8, 2008, from http://studymore.org.uk/01.htm

Roberts, A. (1981c). Glossary – Mental health history words. Retrieved May 15, 2009, from http://www.mdx.ac.uk/www/study/mhhglo.htm

Roberts, A. (1981d/1666). Retrieved May 15, 2009, from http://studymore.org.uk/mhhtim.htm#1666

Roberts, A. (2008). Email. In G. Morgan (Ed.) (Email ed.). London.

Rodwell, C. M. (1996). An analysis of the concept of empowerment. *Journal of Advanced Nursing, 23*(2), 305–313.

Royal-College-of-Psychiatrists'-Spirituality-and-Psychiatry-Special-Interest--Group-Executive-Committee. (2010). Spirituality and mental health [Electronic Version]. Retrieved May 24, 2011, from http://www.rcpsych.ac.uk/mentalhealthinfo/treatments/spirituality.aspx

Rush, B. (2004). Mental health service user involvement in England: Lessons from history. *Journal of Psychiatric & Mental Health Nursing, 11*(3), 313–318.

Russell, D. C. (2013). *The Cambridge companion to virtue ethics.* Cambridge/New York: Cambridge University Press.

Ruth, T. (2007, November 21). Interviewer: G.Morgan, Advocacy interviews, Ivs-RT. London.

Ryan, T., Pritchard, J., & NetLibrary, I. (Eds.). (2004). *Good practice in adult mental health.* London/Philadelphia: Jessica Kingsley Publishers.

Sam, U. (2008, February 13). Interviewer: G.Morgan, Advocacy interviews, Ivs-SU. London.

Sam, U. (2008). *Personal communication*. In G. Morgan (Ed.). London.

Sang, B., & O'Brien, J. (1984). *Advocacy: The UK and American experiences*. London: King Edward's Hospital Fund for London.

Sarah, G, & Karim, H. (2008, December 4). Interviewer: G.Morgan, Advocacy interviews, Ivs-SG/KH. London.

Schön, D. (1983). *The reflective practitioner: How professionals think in action*. London: Maurice Temple Smith Ltd..

Scottish-Independent-Advocacy-Alliance. (2010). *Independent advocacy: A guide for commissioners*. Edinburgh: Scottish Independent Advocacy Alliance.

Scourfield, P. (2007a). A commentary on the emerging literature on advocacy for older people. *Quality in Ageing, 8*(4), 18–27.

Scourfield, P. (2008). Going for brokerage: A task of 'independent support' or social work? *British Journal of Social Work*, bcn141.

Sellman, D. (2000). Alasdair MacIntyre and the professional practice of nursing. *Journal of Nursing Philosophy, 1*(1), 26–33.

Sennett, R. (1998). *The corrosion of character: The personal consequences of work in the new capitalism*. New York: Norton.

Shakespeare, T. (2006). *Disability rights and wrongs*. London/New York: Routledge.

Shepherd, N. (2009). *Trying to be a Christian: A qualitative study of young people's participation in two Youth Ministry projects*. Unpublished Ph.D., King's College London, London.

Silverman, D. (2006). *Interpreting qualitative data: Methods for analyzing talk, text, and interaction*. London/Thousand oaks: SAGE.

Sim, A. J., & Mackay, R. (1997). Advocacy in the UK. *Practice, 9*(2), 5–12.

Sines, D. (1995). Empowering consumers: The caring challenge. *British Journal of Nursing, 4*(8), 445–448.

Singh, I., Roberts, N., Irving, R., & Singh, N. (2013). Compassion, care, dignity and respect: The NHS needs a culture change. *British Journal of Hospital Medicine, 74*(3), 124–125.

Slote, M. (1997). Virtue ethics. In M. Baron, P. Pettit, & M. Slote (Eds.), *Three methods of ethics: A debate* (pp. 175–194). Oxford: Blackwell.

Smith, P. (1992). *The emotional labour of nursing: Its impact on the interpersonal relations, management and the educational environment in nursing*. Basingstoke: Macmillan Education.

Smith, R., Ford, V., Thomas, P., & Bracken, P. (2000). Value of advocacy. *Psychiatr Bull, 24*(1), 30b–331.

Sokol, D. (2009). The value of hospital chaplains. Retrieved April 23, 2009, from http://news.bbc.co.uk/1/hi/health/7990099.stm

Sperry, L. (2012). *Spirituality in clinical practice: Theory and practice of spiritually oriented psychotherapy.* New York: Routledge.

Stephenson, J. (2012). Wellbeing measure 'will boost health investment' [Electronic Version]. *Health Service Journal,* from http://www.hsj.co.uk/news/wellbeing-measure-will-boost-health-investment/5047492.article

Strauss, A. L., & Corbin, J. M. (1998). *Basics of qualitative research: Techniques and procedures for developing grounded theory.* Thousand Oaks: Sage.

Sumner, E. C. (1993). Subscribing to psychiatric history. *History of Psychiatry, 4*(15), 395–412.

Swift, C., Chaplaincy-Leaders-Forum, & National Equality and Health Inequalities Team, N.-E. (2015). *NHS Chaplaincy guidelines 2015, promoting excellence in pastoral, spiritual and religious care.* London: NHS England.

Swinton, J. (2001). Spirituality and the lives of people with learning disabilities. *Updates: Spirituality and Learning Disabilities, 3*(6), 1–4.

Swinton, J., & Mowat, H. (2006). *Practical theology and qualitative research.* London: SCM.

Swinton, J., Mowat, H., & Baines, S. (2011). Whose story am i? Redescribing profound intellectual disability in the kingdom of God. *Health Journal of Religion, Disability and Health, 15*(1), 5–19.

Taylor, C. (1989). *Sources of the self: The making of modern identity.* Cambridge, MA: Harvard University Press.

Tew, J. (2003). Emancipatory research in mental health. In S. Cochrane (Ed.), *SPN paper 4: Where you stand affects your point of view. Emancipatory approaches to mental health research notes from SPN study day: 12 June 2003* (pp. 24–27). London: Social Perspectives Network.

Tew, J. (2008). Researching in partnership: Reflecting on a collaborative study with mental health service users into the impact of compulsion. *Qualitative Social Work, 7*(3), 271–287.

The-American-Heritage-dictionary. (Ed.) (2000). Boston: Houghton Mifflin.

The-College-of-Social-Work/Skills-for-Care. (2014). Fact sheet overview of the care act [Electronic Version]. Retrieved September 22, 2015, from http://www.skillsforcare.org.uk/Document-library/Standards/Care-Act/learning-and-development/introduction-and-overview/care-act-overview-fact-sheet.pdf

The-Lord-Chancellor. (2007). *Mental Capacity Act 2005 Code of Practice.* Retrieved January 19, 2013, from http://webarchive.nationalarchives.gov.uk/+/http://www.dca.gov.uk/legal-policy/mental-capacity/mca-cp.pdf

Thomason, C. (1987). *Advocacy and the development of community care.* Canterbury: University of Kent/PSSRU.

Thompson, R. (2008). Advocating beyond the institution. *Learning Disability Today, 34*(3), 175–180.

Tracy, D. (1996). *Blessed rage for order: The new pluralism in theology: with a new preface.* Chicago: University of Chicago Press.

Traustadóttir, R. (2006). Learning about self-advocacy from life history: A case study from the United States. *British Journal of Learning Disabilities, 34*(3), 175–180.

Tryon, T. (1689). *A treatise of dreams & visions: Wherein the causes, natures, and uses of nocturnal representations, and the communications both of good and evil angels, as also departed souls, to mankinde are theosophically unfolded, that is according to the word of God, and the harmony of created beeing: To which is added, a discourse of the causes, natures, and cure of phrensie, madness or distraction.* London: publisher not identified.

Tudor, K. (1996). *Mental health promotion: Paradigms and practice.* London/New York: Routledge.

Tuke, S. (1813). *Description of the retreat: An institution near York for insane persons of the Society of Friends; containing an account of its origin and progress, the modes of treatment and a statement of cases.* York: printed for W. Alexander, [etc.].

Turner, P. (2007). Caring for the 'Whole Person': Spiritual aspects of care. In J. Brown & P. Libberton (Eds.), *Principles of professional studies in nursing* (pp. 96–110). New York: Palgrave Macmillan.

Turner, B. (2010). *The new Blackwell companion to the sociology of religion.* Malden: Wiley-Blackwell.

Tyler, A. (2010). *Noah's compass.* London: Vintage.

UKAN. (2006). Retrieved February 9, 2008, from http://www.u-kan.co.uk/about.html

Vaartio, H., Leino-Kilpi, H., Salantera, S., & Suominen, T. (2006). Nursing advocacy: How is it defined by patients and nurses, what does it involve and how is it experienced? *Scandinavian Journal of Caring Sciences, 20*(3), 282–292.

Vanier, J. (2008). *Jean Vanier: Essential writings.* New York: Orbis Books.

Walk, A. (1961). The history of mental nursing: The presidential address at the one hundred and twentieth annual meeting of the royal medico-psychological association held at Cane Hill Hospital, 13 July, 1960. *Journal of Mental Science, 107*(446), 1–17.

Walker, A. (2003). *Recovering deep church: Theological and ecclesial renewal.* King's College London.

Walker, A., & Bretherton, L. (Eds.). (2007). *Remembering our future: Explorations in deep church.* London: Paternoster.

Wallcraft, J. (2003). User focused research. In S. Cochrane (Ed.), *SPN Paper 4: Where you stand affects your point of view. Emancipatory approaches to mental health research notes from SPN Study Day: 12 June 2003.* London: Social Perspectives Network.

Ward, P. (1995). *The church and youth ministry.* Oxford/Sutherland: Lynx Communications/Albatross Books.

Ward, D., & Mullender, A. (1991). Empowerment and oppression: An indissoluble pairing for contemporary social work. *Critical Social Policy, 11*(32), 21–30.

Watt, E. (1997). An exploration of the way in which the concept of patient advocacy is perceived by registered nurses working in an acute care hospital. *International Journal of Nursing Practice, 3*(2), 119–127.

Wells, S. (2007). Dementia advocacy. *Working with Older People: Community Care Policy & Practice, 11*(1), 25–27.

Whyte, J. (1987). Practical theology. In A. Campbell (Ed.), *A dictionary of pastoral care* (pp. 212–213). London: SPCK.

Wilkinson, R. G., & Pickett, K. (2010). *The spirit level: Why equality is better for everyone.* London/New York: Penguin Books.

Willard, C. (1996). The nurse's role as patient advocate: Obligation or imposition? [Article]. *Journal of Advanced Nursing, 24*(1), 60–66.

Williams, B. (1985). *Ethics and the limits of philosophy.* Cambridge, MA: Harvard University Press.

Williams, R. (2010, September 14). 'Mate crime' fears for people with learning disabilities. Learning disabled people living in the community are increasingly finding themselves the victims of so-called mate crime. *The Guardian.*

Williams, P., & Shoultz, B. (1982). *We can speak for ourselves: Self-Advocacy by mentally handicapped people.* London: Souvenir Press.

Winston, B. E., & Tucker, P. A. (2011). The beatitudes as leadership virtues. *The Journal of Virtues and Leadership, 2*(1), 15–29.

Wistow, G., & Barnes, M. (1993). User involvement and community care. *Public Administration, 71*(Winter), 279–299.

Wolfensberger, W. (1972). *The principle of normalization in human services.* Toronto: National Institute on Mental Retardation.

Wolfensberger, W. (1977). *A balanced multi-component advocacy/protection schema.* Downsview: Association Resources Division, Canadian Association for the Mentally Retarded.

Wolfensberger, W. (1995). A brief outline of some of th emost important concepts and assumptions underlying citizen advocacy. *The Citizen Advocacy Forum, 5*(January–March), 16–21.

Wolfensberger, W. (2001a). The good life for mentally retarded persons. *Journal of Religion, Disability & Health, 4*(2-3), 103–109.

Wolfensberger, W. (2001b). The normative lack of Christian communality in local congregations as the central obstacle to a proper relationship with needy members. *Journal of Religion, Disability & Health, 4*(2-3), 111–126.

Wolfteich, C. E. (2012). Spirituality. In B. J. Miller-McLemore (Ed.), *The Wiley-Blackwell companion to practical theology* (pp. 328–336). Malden: Wiley-Blackwell.

Wright, N. T. (1992). *The new testament and the people of God.* Minneapolis: Fortress Press.

Wright, T. (2011). Review. *Thresholds: Counselling with spirit, Summer 2011.*

Wright, A. (2012). *Christianity and critical realism: Ambiguity, truth, and theological literacy.* London/New York: Routledge.

Xiaoyan, B., & Yow-wu, B. W. (2008). Development and psychometric evaluation of the instrument: Attitude toward patient advocacy. *Research in Nursing & Health, 31*(1), 63–75.

Yeadon, C. (1990, October 6). *Citizen advocacy principles and peversions.* Paper presented at the World Citizen Advocacy Congress, Lincoln, Nebraska.

Yin, R. K. (2006). *Case study research: Design and methods.* Thousand Oaks: Sage.

Zablon, V. (2008, September 19). Interviewer: G.Morgan, Advocacy interviews, Ivs-ZV. London.

Index

Note: Page numbers followed by 'n' denote notes

© The Author(s) 2017   **267**
G. Morgan, *Independent Advocacy and Spiritual Care*,
DOI 10.1057/978-1-137-53125-4

The manufacturer's authorised representative in the EU is Springer
Nature Customer Service Centre GmbH, Europaplatz 3, 69115 Heidelberg,
Germany. If you have any concerns regarding our products, please
contact ProductSafety@springernature.com

Printed and bound by CPI Group (UK) Ltd, Croydon, CR0 4YY
23/04/2026
02095587-0008